Computers in
Nursing's

Nurses' Guide
to the Internet

3RD EDITION

About the Author

Leslie H. Nicoll

Leslie H. Nicoll, PhD, MBA, RN, is the Editor-in-Chief of *Computers in Nursing*, the only international peer-reviewed journal in nursing that focuses exclusively on computers, informatics, and technology, published by Lippincott Williams & Wilkins, Philadelphia, Pennsylvania. In addition, Dr. Nicoll is a Research Associate Professor in the College of Nursing and Health Professions and Senior Research Associate in the Edmund S. Muskie School of Public Service, both at the University of Southern Maine, Portland, Maine. In this role, Dr. Nicoll provides research consultation and technical assistance to a wide variety of individuals and organizations. Clinically, Dr. Nicoll is active in the hospice and palliative care community in the state of Maine. She has served as Principal Investigator for HAPCEN: Hospice and Palliative Care Education Network, funded by the National Cancer Institute from 1995-1998. Currently, she is a partner on a statewide grant on Community-State Partnerships in End-of-Life Care, funded by the Robert Wood Johnson Foundation (1999-2001). Dr. Nicoll is an active member of Sigma Theta Tau International. She has served on several international committees and is currently a member of the Distinguished Lecturer Program and a collateral reviewer for research grants. Dr. Nicoll is a graduate of Russell Sage College (BS, Nursing), the University of Illinois (MS, Nursing Sciences), and Case Western Reserve University (PhD, Nursing). As a Commonwealth Fund Executive Nurse Fellow, she pursued MBA study at the Whittemore School of Business and Economics, University of New Hampshire, graduating in 1991. Dr. Nicoll is happily married to Tony Jendrek and is the mother of two wonderful children, Lance and Hannah.

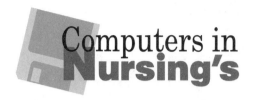

Computers in Nursing's

Nurses' Guide
to the Internet

3RD EDITION

Leslie H. Nicoll, PhD, MBA, RN

Editor-in-Chief, *Computers in Nursing*
College of Nursing and Health Professions
E.S. Muskie School of Public Service
University of Southern Maine
Portland, Maine

Lippincott
Philadelphia · New York · Baltimore

Acquisitions Editor: Sandra Kasko
Project Editor: Debra Schiff
Senior Production Manager: Helen Ewan
Production Coordinator: Patricia McCloskey
Design Coordinator: Brett MacNaughton
Interior Designer: Holly Reid McLaughlin
Cover Designer: Tom Jackson
Manufacturing Manager: William Alberti

Edition 3rd

9   8   7   6   5   4   3   2

Library of Congress Cataloging-in-Publication Data

Nicoll, Leslie H.
Computers in nursing's nurses' guide to the Internet / Leslie H. Nicoll.--3rd ed.
    p. ; cm.
Includes bibliographical references and index.
ISBN 0-7817-2459-7 (alk. paper)
    1. Nursing–Computer network resources. 2. Internet. 3. Nursing informatics. I. Title:
Nurses's guide to the Internet. II Title.
    [DNLM: 1. Internet. 2. Nursing. 3. Information Systems. WY 26.5 N645c 2001]
RT50.5 .N53 2001
025.06'61073—dc21
                                                                    00-058642

Care has been taken to confirm the accuracy of the information presented and to describe generally accepted practices. However, the authors, editors, and publisher are not responsible for errors or omissions or for any consequences from application of the information in this book and make no warranty, express or implied, with respect to the content of the publication.

The authors, editors, and publisher have exerted every effort to ensure that drug selection and dosage set forth in this text are in accordance with the current recommendations and practice at the time of publication. However, in view of ongoing research, changes in government regulations, and the constant flow of information relating to drug therapy and drug reactions, the reader is urged to check the package insert for each drug for any change in indications and dosage and for added warnings and precautions. This is particularly important when the recommended agent is a new or infrequently employed drug.

Some drugs and medical devices presented in this publication have Food and Drug Administration (FDA) clearance for limited use in restricted research settings. It is the responsibility of the health care provider to ascertain the FDA status of each drug or device planned for use in his or her clinical practice.

Preface and Acknowledgments

I have been online for almost 15 years now. On one hand, 15 years is not that long, but when I look at the changes that have occurred in computers and technology, it seems like a lifetime. My introduction to the online world came in 1987. I was attending the Sigma Theta Tau (International Honor Society of Nursing) Biennial Convention in San Francisco. In the Exhibit Hall was a staff member from the National Library of Medicine, demonstrating GratefulMed. GratefulMed was a software program that allowed an individual to search the databases, such as MEDLINE, of the National Library of Medicine. At first, I was totally dismayed when I saw this program. I had defended my dissertation just 3 weeks before the conference. How I could have used this program while I was writing the proposal, conducting the research, and writing the final paper that became my dissertation! I quickly realized, however, that even though I had finished that component of my professional education, I knew that acquiring literature resources would continue to be part of my professional life.

I came home from that conference, ordered the software, and became connected to the online world. Although I had had a computer on my desk since 1983, this was the first time I was able to reach out, connect to another computer, and obtain information that was transmitted to me instantly. That first connection was the beginning of a profound change in how I carry out my day-to-day work.

The intervening years have brought many more changes. My first modem was a "zippy" 1200 baud; now I connect to the Internet through a high-speed cable modem connected to a cable television line. If I am on the road, I can also connect using a modem and cellular phone (no more outrageous long-distance charges in hotel rooms for me!). GratefulMed has morphed from an early DOS program, through Windows, and now is available exclusively on the Internet (http://igm.nlm.nih.gov); it is totally free to users who search through the Internet. Remember 10-megabyte hard drives? I am sitting here with a 6-gigabyte hard drive installed in a laptop computer that weighs less than 5 pounds!

But the biggest change of all is the world of the Internet and the World Wide Web. Pictures have replaced text; videos, music, and more have brought my computer to life. Information pours through cyberspace and into my machine at a rate at which it is almost impossible to keep pace. It is clear that the explosive growth of the Internet is the most exciting new communication opportunity seen in my lifetime. At least, so far. Who knows where technology will take us next? When I think of the changes that have occurred in just 15 years, it boggles my mind to imagine what technology will offer me in 2015.

Through these past 15 years of online exploration and investigation, I have become very comfortable with the Internet and the resources it has to offer. When I need information, I turn to the Internet first. This is true in my personal, as well as my professional, life. I shop online and find goods and services that are not available in Maine. A few years ago I purchased Pergo ® flooring online from a supplier in California; even though it is sold all over now, I am convinced that I was the first person in Maine to have Pergo ® in my house. When my son needs to do research for a school paper, he turns to the Internet. My daughter, at 9 years of age, wields the mouse like an accomplished chef with a knife as she surfs from place to place. Even my husband, reluctant at first, has become a savvy Internet traveler.

As Editor-in-Chief of *Computers in Nursing*, nurses have contacted me regularly to ask questions about Internet resources, information, or just how to get connected. I have learned that there are many nurses who are taking their first tentative steps toward discovering the world of online information and resources. They are enthusiastic, but not sure where to begin. I have received repeated requests for information on sources and sites that would be of particular interest to nurses. People also asked me for suggestions of a useful guide or book that they could use to get started. After doing some research, I realized that such a guide did not exist. Thus, the idea for the *Nurses' Guide to the Internet* was born.

The first edition of this *Guide* was published in 1996; the second edition came out 24 months later in 1998. With both editions, I received a high level of positive feedback from readers. "Simple," "concise," "easy-to-read," "you make it clear for a novice" were some of the comments I received. With each revision, I have taken my cues from you, my readers, and have considered your needs and wishes with each edition of this book. As a matter of fact, I believe I have come to know my readers very well. Over the past 5 years, I have been asked to speak at numerous conferences, workshops, and educational seminars on the topic of the Internet.[1] I

---

[1] I thoroughly enjoy opportunities to speak to nurses and other health care professionals about the Internet and other aspects of informatics in health care. If you are planning a seminar or workshop and would be interested in having me present, please feel free to contact me directly at *LNICOLL@maine.rr.com* or by telephone at 207-415-1590.

have spoken to audiences with as few as 10 participants or as many as 1,000. Whenever I begin, I ask people to identify themselves as novice, intermediate, or expert. Almost without exception, the audience divides themselves fairly evenly into novice and intermediate, with only a tiny percentage (often just one or two people) calling themselves expert. (As an aside, I am no longer surprised when the self-identified expert many times asks some of the most basic questions during the session! This only reinforces to me that there is so much to learn and know about the Internet, that even experts, such as myself, often have gaps in knowledge about the technology.) My presentation experience, as well as e-mail communication with many of my readers, has reinforced that you want an easily accessible, hands-on guide that addresses the basics of getting online, e-mail, searching, and navigating the World Wide Web, along with recommendations of useful sites for professional nurses. With those guidelines in mind, I am pleased to present you with a completely updated, revised, expanded, and overhauled third edition of *Computers in Nursing's Nurses' Guide to the Internet.*

Although the content has been revised from top to bottom, some things have not changed. Just as with the first two editions, the information included in this Internet tour guide has been selected with an eye to efficient and rewarding professional Internet travel. The book is designed for nurses who have a desire and interest to "get on the Internet" but do not know where to start. In the book I provide different types of resources: a general overview and user's guide that provides basic information (Part I, Chapters 1 through 5) and an alphabetical directory of more than 510 sites, with addresses, contact information, and descriptions of each one (Part II). At the back of the book is a comprehensive, cross-referenced index to the sites in the book as well as an index to the text in the first five chapters. Every site has been visited, every mailing list has been subscribed to—I have done my very best to bring you the most complete and current information possible. I hope that you find it useful in your work or maybe even *your* personal life.

Once major change in this edition is the content included in Chapter 4. Much of what is discussed in that chapter—e-commerce, Internet telephony, synchronous chatting—did not exist (or existed in a limited form) when the second edition was written two years ago. Although the "granddaddy" of Internet chatting, IRC, did exist at that time, it was difficult to use, especially for the novice. New programs, such as ICQ and Instant Messenger (from America Online), have made online chatting as commonplace as talking on the telephone. Recognizing these trends, I have expanded the book to include this new chapter with discussion of these resources, and more. Although online shopping may not be directly related to professional nursing, I have been asked the question enough by nurses that I believe including this content is essential for this new edition.

This book is a natural outgrowth of the work I do as Editor-in-Chief of *Computers in Nursing.* It is a pleasure to have the strong support of my publisher at Lippincott Williams & Wilkins, Sandra Kasko, and her talented and capable staff. I also appreciate the contributions of my former publisher, Lisa Marshall, and I am grateful for her assistance with this edition on a freelance basis. It is exciting to have a variety of methods with which to deliver the *Computers in Nursing* message to nurses around the world and the support of Lippincott to deliver that message. The print version of the journal, with its peer-reviewed articles, research reports, news, and reviews continues to break ground in the world of nursing informatics. This book, in combination with the journal, and information available online at NursingCenter.com, provides an array of useful resources to meet the computer information needs of nurses in all settings.

Earlier I mentioned my personal life. There are some very important people in my life who deserve my deepest thanks for their continuing and unending support—all of my family, but most especially my wonderful husband Tony and my loving and sweet children, Lance and Hannah. They are very proud of their mother and I am very proud of them! Since the second edition of the book came out, my elderly cats, Pookah and Bandit, have gone to the Rainbow Bridge to join their mother and friends, but we are still delighted with the newest member of our family, a retired racing greyhound named Jessie (check out the "Dogs" section of the Index). All of my family, human and canine, help to bring a balance to my busy and sometimes overly hectic life. Thanks to all of you—and thank you, too, dear reader, for your support of my professional work.

Leslie H. Nicoll, PhD, MBA, RN
Westbrook, Maine
October 2000

Contents

PART I

INTRODUCTION AND OVERVIEW OF INTERNET TRAVEL

CHAPTER 1

■■

Surfing Is Great . . . If You Are on Vacation

HELLO, TRAVELER . . .

Welcome to the world of Internet travel. I have written this book to assist you as you begin your Internet journey. I have designed it to be a travel guide. Why did I decide to use that analogy? Well, I am assuming that if you are looking at this book, you have an interest in exploring the Internet. If so, you are about to embark on an exciting trip. Whenever I take a trip, I find that if I read a travel guide beforehand, I have a more successful adventure. But I bring the book with me, so that I know where the good sights are and how to find the best restaurants. I have discovered that Internet travel is no different. Although it is possible to dive right in and begin exploring, if you want to find specific material or particular types of information, your trip will be more rewarding with a handy travel guide. Thus, this book.

Lots of people talk about "surfing the Web" (short for World Wide Web or WWW) or "surfing the 'net" (short for "Internet"). Surfing is great, if you are on vacation. In fact, I have been known to while away many hours, surfing through the world of cyberspace. But there are times when it is necessary to put fun aside and buckle down to get some work done. Often, that work will require acquiring information and resources from the Internet. In that case, you are on a "professional trip," not vacation. In writing this guide, I am assuming that you are on either a business trip or a professional journey. Therefore, the information I have opted to include has been selected with an eye to professional, not vacation, travel. There are lots of Internet guides for the vacationing Internet surfer. There are not as many that deal with business travel for the professional nurse. This guide has been written to fill that gap.

A FEW ASSUMPTIONS

I am presuming several things about you, my reader. First, you are a nurse or, perhaps, a student studying to become a nurse. Either way, this book has been written with nurses in mind. Although other health professionals are welcome to read and use this book, I have geared the information in this guide to the needs of the working professional nurse. I know that nurses work in a variety of settings, doing a wide range of activities, in many different specialty areas. Using my experience, expertise, and interests, I have sought to include information that will be useful for the world of nurses with their wide range of professional pursuits.

Second, you are busy. Every day I experience the feeling of too much work and too few hours in which to accomplish it all. I imagine you have the same frustration. As you start on your Internet journey, I am assuming that you do not have time to waste. In fact, many people cite their lack of time as a barrier to becoming acquainted with the Internet—they believe that the time spent learning will not be rewarded with acquisition of useful information. Thus, I have tried to be concise to help you get started in a timely and efficient manner. Similarly, I have selected sites and resources to be useful and of interest to you as a busy professional. I have tried, as much as possible, to separate "the wheat from the chaff."

Nothing is more frustrating than hearing about a great resource on the Internet and then finding out that it has been dismantled, or worse yet, abandoned by its developer. I have endeavored to select sites that are "going concerns," that is, sites that will be around for a while. An emerging phenomenon of the Internet is the fact that just about anybody with access can create a Web page, bulletin board, or discussion group and put it "out there" for anyone else to see, use, or access. Although this explosion of information is exciting, it has also led to lots of sites that are quickly rendered obsolete and never updated. Although I cannot guarantee that every Internet site included in the "Directory of Sites" will, in fact, be active when you go to access it, I have tried to select sites that appear to have a reasonable chance of survival on the Internet. In this way, this guide will help you to not waste too much time by visiting sites that no longer exist.

Third, you are a professional. As a professional, you want and need accurate, up-to-date information for your nursing work but you also realize that you have a responsibility to assess the information that you obtain from whatever source. I am assuming that you use your critical thinking skills to verify all information you gather for your professional practice. Information obtained from the Internet is no different. For this guide, in selecting sites, I have chosen those that appear to be accurate, documented, updated, and contain useful information. I have done this by verifying dates when sites were created or updated, investigating the credentials of the site developer, and reviewing the material contained at the site. However, information on the Internet changes with the speed of light (or typing fingers on the keyboard). Therefore, even though I have done a preliminary screening, you must exercise your professional responsibility and personally assess information that you obtain from the Internet. As you visit sites listed in this guide, you will have the benefit of my assessment. But information may very well have changed from the time I visited the site and the time you do. Keep that in mind and do your own checking. Similarly, once you become familiar with Internet travel, you will be visiting sites that are not listed in these pages. You will need to develop your own criteria for evaluation, so that you can be assured that the information is truly useful and accurate for your work. I have included information on evaluation in Chapter 3, but I would still suggest that you use my criteria as a guide. Develop your own criteria for evaluation so that you can be confident in the information that you find.

Fourth, you realize the value of information from a variety of sources. I hope to introduce you to the Internet so that it can become yet another component of your nursing armamentarium. But do not ignore other existing resources, including professional journals, books, libraries, audiovisuals, and publications from professional societies and organizations. The Internet is not the "be all and end all" of information. It is a useful resource and it can bring to your desktop information that previously might have taken you days or weeks to find. Using the Internet can often save you a trip to the library or the cost of an envelope and stamp. But do not be fooled into thinking that all information is available on the Internet. It is not. As you become a seasoned traveler, you'll have a greater appreciation for what can be found where. Then you'll be in the best position to use your information resources wisely.

Finally, as a nurse, I believe you are adventurous, tenacious, creative, and patient. I have found that these characteristics are often the defining feature of a successful nurse. To be an effective Internet traveler, you need to apply these same elements to your Internet journey. This book is a starting point, but you will encounter many situations in which you are not finding the information or resources that you are seeking. If something is not working, think to yourself: "What does it take to solve this problem?" Do you need to try a little harder (tenacity), try a little longer (patience), or approach the problem in a different way (creativity)? I have found that each Internet stumbling block requires its own unique brand of problem solving. Keep that in mind so that you can enjoy your journey and not become frustrated when the answer is not immediate.

USING THIS GUIDE

As you begin your journey, I plan to offer you some keys to success that can make your trip more rewarding and productive. To meet this goal, I have organized this book in the manner of a traditional travel guide, with two major parts and a traditional index. Part I (which you are currently reading) includes a general overview of Internet travel. In the following chapter, I have included some "basic travel tips"—getting online, necessary equipment, information on Internet addresses and language, and glossaries of helpful terms, abbreviations, and glyphs. The "Site-Seeing" guide in Chapter 3 includes an overview of the sites available on the Internet, a few caveats about what to expect and what not to expect, tips for effective searching, and information on making the transition from Internet traveler to Internet explorer. Chapter 4 includes some diversions for your traveling experience: shopping online, discussion groups, Internet telephony, and more. The user's guide for the "Directory of Sites" comprises Chapter 5.

Part II is the core of the book, "The Directory of Sites." This is your roadmap for your journey. In a traditional travel guide, this section would be the hotel and restaurant listings; in this book, the directory includes information on World Wide Web (WWW) sites and Listservs, with descriptions at each entry and contact information when available. In the back of the book is a detailed, cross-referenced index that will point you to the information you are seeking in the Directory. The "Directory of Sites" in Part II is arranged in strict alphabetical order, not by topic or specialty area. Listing the sites alphabetically facilitates finding a particular entry when you know it is there, but the alphabetical format makes it more difficult to find related areas of information. Of course, you can just browse through the Directory and read the entries at your leisure. But if you want to find specific information—say, all the sites related to "cancer"—then be sure to use the Index. The Index will point you to *all* of the entries in the Directory related to a particular topic area. So don't ignore the Index; in some ways, it is the most important part of the book.

Enough introduction—let's get started on our trip!

CHAPTER 2

■■

Basic Travel Tips

THE FIRST STEP: GETTING ONLINE

In the real world, the first step in any trip is to figure out how to get there: by plane, train, bus, or car. Internet travel is no different. Your first step in Internet travel is to get connected, electronically, to the Internet world.

If you are connecting to the Internet solely through work or school, then you might not need to consider issues of hardware, software, and Internet connection. Someone else will have made these decisions, and you will be using equipment that is set up and ready to go. But maybe you do not have access through work—or you do, but you also want to be able to connect from home. If that is the case, read on. There are some issues you need to consider and important decisions you need to make.

Determining the type of Internet connection that is right for you requires some thought. Everyone immediately thinks hardware (what type of computer) and software are the primary concerns. However, your first step should be a quick assessment of your personal needs. You will be paying for an Internet connection, one way or another. Therefore, do not buy and pay for services you will not use. Consider your personal or professional communication requirements. Some questions to consider are the following:

- Do you want to transfer files between computer systems throughout the world?
- Do you need to browse other computer systems such as those maintained by university libraries?
- Are you interested in exploring the new multimedia technologies that have recently flooded the World Wide Web (WWW)?
- Are you interested in sending electronic mail (e-mail) to friends and colleagues?

- What is your practice area? Are you practicing in a specialty area that requires up-to-the minute practice information?
- Are you a student or nurse author, writing papers and manuscripts and needing literature resources?
- Are you a researcher and need access to data types and sources available online?
- Are you a student interested in taking courses online?

You may very well come up with a list of your own questions that will require some thought. Take your time and envision how you will be using your Internet access, because the answers to these questions will help you determine the type and kind of services that you need from an Internet provider.

Connecting to the Internet requires a number of components, with several options, depending on the depth of service you need. The most useful approach is to try to find a variety of components delivered in one package, not multiple options for each. Even if you think you want access just for e-mail, it will not be long before you discover that you want some information that is available on the WWW. Therefore, you'll be better prepared if, at the outset, you try to establish a connection that will give you the greatest flexibility in adding or deleting services as you need them. More detail on options that are available will be presented later. For now, let's start at the beginning: hardware, software, and Internet Service Providers (ISPs) for Internet connectivity.

HARDWARE

Computer

There is not a computer being sold today that does not have the necessary components for accessing the Internet. The Internet has become so popular that all new computer buyers have this as a requirement, not an option. Does that mean you need to go out and buy a new machine? Not necessarily. Even an older personal computer can connect to the Internet without too much trouble. But the type of Internet services you can access will depend, to some extent, on how much computing power you have. An older computer with a slow modem will work just fine for e-mail or file transfer, but to really travel on the WWW, a much higher end computer is required.

The WWW is made up of multimedia resources. WWW browsers, such as Microsoft's Internet Explorer or Netscape's Communicator, are based on graphical user interfaces. In other words, you see pictures, graphics, video and movies, hear music, and read text. These multimedia features require a fast microprocessor, a good-sized hard drive, and sufficient amounts of random access memory to run properly on computers with either Windows or Macintosh operating systems.

If you are buying a new computer, take the time to do your homework. Read magazine articles in computer magazines such as *PC World* or *Byte*, and consult with your friends, colleagues, and knowledgeable sales people to determine the best system for your needs. Remember this computer-buying truism as you begin shopping: buy the computer with the most computing power (microprocessor, random access memory, storage, video, and so on) that you can afford. Although it is often true that the computer you buy today will be obsolete tomorrow, you can do your best to stay ahead of technology by buying at the higher end, whenever possible.

If you are a total computer novice, you might want to spend some time using another computer to find out what you like and what works well for you. For example, if you take a college course you may be able to use the computers in the college lab. There may be a mix of computers, including Macintoshes and personal computers (PCs) with Microsoft Windows. Which do you prefer? If you are not a novice, use your prior computer experience as a guide to what you should buy.

Necessary Equipment for Getting Connected

No matter what kind of computer you have—desktop or laptop, Macintosh or PC—your next step is to obtain the necessary equipment to make a connection to the Internet. Just a few years ago, you had essentially two choices: through a local area network (LAN) or by dial-in access through a telephone modem. New options, including cable modems and TV Internet devices, have recently become available.

NETWORKS

Most institutions connect to the Internet using a local area network. In this setup, each individual computer has a network card inside the machine, which allows the computer to connect to a local server. Each computer has a unique Internet protocol (IP) address. The local server provides the connection to a larger area network, often known as a wide area network (WAN). It is through these connections that you are able, from your desk, to communicate with computers all over the world. The actual technical configuration varies from institution to institution, but the concept is the same for any group of networked computers. The network connection is made through high-speed, fiber optic connections; you are not connecting through a telephone line.

Network connections are great: they are fast and reliable and provide almost immediate access to the resources of the WWW. However, networks are expensive to set up and require a high level of technical service to maintain. A network connection from home is not a realistic option for the vast majority of people. Therefore, if you are investigating your home Internet connection, you will need to look at other options, a discussion of which follows.

MODEMS

The most popular way to connect to the Internet via a home or office stand-alone computer is through a modem. Although there are other ways to connect, industry estimates still have more than 90% of users accessing the Internet using a modem. A *modem* is used to transmit digital information from a computer through ordinary phone lines to a network provider or Internet access provider. All modems work basically the same way and are generally packaged with the communication software needed to make them work. An internal modem fits into a slot inside the computer, whereas an external modem sits outside the computer with its own power supply and connects to the serial port on a PC or to the modem port on a Macintosh. For portable computers, there are modems that are as small as credit cards and fit in a PC card slot on the laptop. The type you select can be a personal choice or may be dictated by your computer's configuration. As with buying a computer, if you do not own a modem, it is wise to consult knowledgeable friends or salespeople. Modem reviews and information on what to buy are also available online: check sites such as ZDNet (www.zdnet.com) or Cnet (www.cnet.com).

Although there are many aspects to selecting a modem, perhaps the most important in terms of Internet access is speed. Modem speeds are reported in kbps, or kilobits per second. What is a kilobit? The letter k stands for the Greek prefix *kilo,* meaning 1,000. (There's also m for *mega,* or million.) Bits per second—the rate at which a modem or network transmits data—is commonly abbreviated as bps. With an uppercase K instead, the rate refers to kilobytes, rather than kilobits.

So what's a byte? Every individual character a computer contains, displays, transmits, or receives is called a byte, and each byte is composed of eight data bits. So when you see a modem rated at 33.6k or 56.6k, what you're actually seeing is a device that can transmit 33,600 or 56,600 bits of data—or the equivalent of one to two pages of text—per second. (Modem manufacturers often abbreviate 56.6 kbps as 56k.) The current standard for modem speed is 56k. If you are shopping for a new modem, this is what will be available to you. If you have an older modem in your computer, it may be running at a slower speed, such as 33.6 kpbs or even 14.4 kbps. Obviously, the slower the modem, the slower your Internet connection will be, which means that Websites, graphics, and files will take longer to load on your screen.

Many modems sold today are fax-modems; in addition to communicating with other computers, you can send and receive faxes from your computer. Most modems come packaged with communication software, such as Bitcom or Procomm, as well as fax software, such as Faxworks or Winfax. If you are in a situation in which you need to buy a separate communication software package, be sure that it will support vt100 terminal emulation and Kermit or Zmodem file transfers. This ensures that your software can "talk" to the mainframe computer with which you'll eventually be communicating.

CABLE MODEMS

Fairly recent innovations are cable modems; at present, these modems have limited availability in the United States, but the market is growing on a daily basis. Industry experts estimate that there are currently around 1 million cable modem subscribers in the US and that number is predicted to triple within the next few years. A cable modem hooks to the cable line used for television, as opposed to the phone line that is used by a traditional modem. The cable modem is an external modem with its own power supply. With a cable modem setup, you will need a network card in the computer (the same type of card used for a network connection). Two connections are made to the modem: the cable line (from the outside) and the network connection from the network card in the computer.

To be able to use a cable modem, you must be in a location that has cable television and offers cable modem service. If the cable line is not available to your home (or office), then obviously you will not be able to make a cable connection. Cable modems are being installed and managed by cable television companies, such as Time Warner. It is not required that you have cable television in order to have a cable modem.

A cable modem has several advantages: it is much faster than a traditional modem; in fact, the speed is similar to that offered by a network connection. You will not be tying up your phone line while you are connected to the Internet. And most companies offer unlimited access—you are not charged by the minute or hour while you are connected. So you can log on and surf to your heart's content without worrying about long-distance phone charges or connect charges through an Internet provider. Prices, although more expensive than providers such as America Online, are generally competitive. The big disadvantage is that you must have cable access and your cable company must offer this service.

DIGITAL SUBSCRIBER LINE

Another newer option is digital subscriber line, or DSL. DSL has been developed by the telephone industry and is a direct competitor with cable modems (which have been developed by the cable television industry). Once again, the major advantage of DSL is high-speed Internet access. Computer geeks like to debate endlessly which is faster: DSL or a cable modem. But the average user (like you and me) would probably be satisfied with either one—and they are both much faster than a traditional modem. The major determinant for most people is not speed but availability. DSL is still in the testing stage in many markets and is not widely available throughout the US. But that is expected to change in the near future, so even if DSL is not available in your town today, it may very well be available tomorrow.

What is DSL? DSL is an always-on Internet connection that ends in a socket on your wall that looks much like a phone socket. At least in the US, the socket is exactly like a phone socket, and for the popular residential DSL, (ADSL), the same house wiring does indeed carry phone and data. DSL is billed per month, usually for a fixed price and, for the majority of providers, for unlimited usage. DSL provides digital access to the Internet over traditional copper phone lines, as opposed to a traditional modem, which uses an analog signal. As with the cable modem, you need specialized equipment and drivers for DSL, but these items are usually provided to you as part of the package when you sign up for DSL service.

DSL is an excellent high-speed alternative to a traditional modem, but you can only take advantage of it if it is available in your community. If my recent experience can be a guide, you will know if it is available: the service will be widely advertised on television, billboards, and in the newspaper. If you are in a DSL-supplied neighborhood, you probably want to investigate this option for your Internet access.

SATELLITE INTERNET ACCESS

Another new option for high-speed access is satellite Internet access. Satellite Internet uses the same type of technology as satellite television reception. Satellite dishes have an advantage over the other technologies discussed here in that they require no infrastructure. If you are in the continental US and have somewhere to put a 21-inch dish facing south, you can get this service. And if you live in a rural area, a satellite dish may be the only high-speed Internet connection available to you. If you already have a satellite, it may be possible to upgrade it to make the Internet connection, although many older satellites are not upgradeable. The computer connects to the Internet through the satellite. A major disadvantage is that the dish can only receive data. You must have a dial-up connection to send. That means you still need a modem, your phone line is still tied up, and you still need an ISP to which you will have to pay a monthly fee. Satellite Internet is supposed to be very fast—faster than a traditional modem or even a cable modem or DSL—although early tests indicate that the service might not quite live up to its claims in this department. It is also very expensive—you need to buy a satellite, pay for installation, and then pay a monthly access charge. If you want to have satellite television, that is a separate charge from the Internet service. Right now, the service is so new and expensive that it is probably not a realistic option for many people. However, as it becomes more popular and widely available, the price will probably drop. For people who live in locales where cable or DSL will never be available, satellite connections may become the only realistic option for fast Internet access.

INTERNET TELEVISION

The final option currently available is Internet television. This is actually quite different from the preceding discussion, because you are not buying a computer. Instead, you buy a device that sits on top of your television and brings the Internet to your home through your television. These devices start at around $100—definitely much less expensive than buying a new computer system. With such a connection, you are able to access the Internet and WWW, send and receive e-mail, and read news groups. Because Internet TV is not a computer, you will not be able to do any other computer activities, such as word processing, desktop publishing, or game playing. The manufacturers of Internet television devices make it clear that these are not a replacement for a home computer. But if you have a computer that is too old for upgrading for Internet access, but not so old that you want to get rid of it, Internet television might be a viable alternative.

A few years ago, many predicted the demise of Internet television, but the technology seems to be thriving. Interestingly, industry experts estimate that 70% of Internet television users do not own a computer and are not planning on acquiring one. Why do they have Internet TV? Primarily for e-mail, it seems.

Many use Internet TV as a way to keep in touch with friends, children, and relatives on an electronic basis.

Making a Connection: The Bridge Between Your Hardware and the Internet

INTERNET SERVICE PROVIDERS

Once you have the proper equipment to make an Internet connection, your next step is to identify a provider for your access. Depending on what type of equipment you have, you may not have to make a decision. If you are connecting to the Internet through a network, then your access issues are solved. Similarly, cable modems, DSL, Internet television, and satellite Internet connections all come with access provision built in. However, if you are one of the vast majority of users who will be connecting through a modem, you need to determine who will be your ISP and how you will access the Internet. In the simplest terms, your ISP will give you a phone number to call and make your Internet connection and provide an e-mail address. If you are connecting through a commercial service, you will pay a monthly fee for this service. You may have other options available to you, such as dialing in through a university, so that your Internet access is free or available for a very minimal fee.

If you are connecting with a modem, you will be dialing in to your provider through a phone line. Therefore, the following issues need to be considered:

- Long-distance versus local call
- Cost of the service
- Availability of connections

Selecting the best service for your needs may be a trade-off between these options.

Long-distance versus local call is a very important consideration. If you must make a long-distance call each time you make a connection, then, obviously, the longer you are online, the more the call will cost. For many people, this process becomes cost prohibitive. For example, if you are a student at a university or college, you may be able to get a university account for Internet access at no charge. But if the number you need to call to make the connection is long distance, it may cost you more in the long run to connect this way. Commercial services, such as America Online or AT&T WorldNet, may be able to provide you with a local number or a toll-free 800 number. So even though you need to pay a monthly fee for the service, it may be cheaper than long-distance charges. The luckiest person is the one who has free university access and a local number to call. For many of us, however, this is just not the case!

A second option is to find a local access provider in your area or one that uses an 800 number for dial-in. Look in the Yellow Pages under "Internet service provider." Service provider rates vary greatly depending on the time of access, speed of access desired, and several other factors. It pays to shop around.

The final point to consider is availability. When your modem makes its call, it will be connecting to another modem at the other end. The number of modems available will determine if you get a connection or a busy signal. One of the advantages that commercial services like to advertise is the high rate of connectivity offered to their customers. If you have a local service provider, a limited number of modems may mean that it is very difficult to get through, especially at peak usage times.

Cost is certainly an important factor, but remember the adage, "You get what you pay for." There are many local ISPs that advertise unlimited monthly access for prices of less than $10 a month. Although that sounds like a great deal, be sure ask what you get for that price. Is there technical support available? How many modems are in their modem pool? The cheapest service may not be the most cost effective in the long run.

Balance all three options together and then shop around to make a final decision. The list of questions in Display 2-1 can be helpful as you investigate different ISPs. Type of call, cost of service, and availability all need to be considered to arrive at a cost-effective and appropriate solution. Keep in mind that your ISP is what will determine your e-mail address (more on this in the next section). I often tell people that changing your e-mail address is like changing your phone number: it can be done, but once you have given your address to all your friends, colleagues, coworkers, and distant relatives, changing it is a bit of a pain in the neck. Therefore, think twice before you sign up with an ISP, because once you are set with an e-mail address, you may not want to change your service. And remember, choosing an ISP is a very individualized decision: what works for you may not be the same option chosen by your neighbor or friend, even if your computing needs are similar.

DISPLAY 2-1. TEN QUESTIONS TO ASK A POTENTIAL ISP

1. Do you have telephone access numbers in my local calling area?
2. Do you offer toll-free access if I am on the road? Is there an extra charge for this? If yes, how much?
3. Do you have a fixed monthly price for unlimited use?
4. Which browser and e-mail reader do you provide?
5. Can I use another browser and e-mail reader of my own choosing?
6. Do you offer more than one e-mail account per subscription? If yes, how many?
7. Do you offer 56 kpbs access? Will your 56 kbps access work with my modem?
8. Do you offer free Web page postings? How many megabytes of server space are available for my own Web page?
9. Do you have toll-free (or local) technical support services? Is technical support available 24 hours a day? If not, what are the hours?
10. Do you have filters to block spam e-mail? (See pg. 33 for a discussion of spam e-mail.)

Software

BROWSER SOFTWARE

The final step in making an Internet connection is software. The software is what will allow you to browse the WWW and send and receive e-mail. Software is what runs on your computer and determines what you see on your monitor. Once you have selected a provider, you need to determine your software needs for both a browser and e-mail. Many providers, such as America Online or Time Warner's Roadrunner cable modem service, include the software as part of the package. But that does not mean you are required to use the browser that they provide. It is possible, for example, to have an account on America Online but use Netscape's Communicator as your browser.

E-MAIL SOFTWARE

The other piece of software you need to acquire is a mail program, which will allow you to send and receive e-mail. Many browser programs have e-mail functions that are built in, but you can also get a stand-alone e-mail application. What are the advantages of the latter? Most stand-alone e-mail programs have additional features, such as advanced filtering options, more sophisticated address books, and the ability to have multiple accounts within one mail program. But the bundled e-mail applications that come with Internet Explorer and Communicator are also quite functional, and most people find they are completely adequate for their needs. The choice is up to you.

Learning to Read the Street Signs

Just like in the real world, the virtual world requires addresses to navigate. To find your way around, you need an understanding of how Internet addresses work.
    Today's Internet uses three addressing schemes:

- Domain name system (DNS)
- E-mail
- Universal resource locator (URL)

Each type of address has a specific purpose. Let us begin with the DNS, which is the foundation of all Internet addresses.
    Every computer node attached to the Internet has a unique numerical address known as an IP (Internet protocol) address. To the computer, it would look something like this: 129.237.28.3. Unfortunately, most of us have trouble remembering numerical sequences, particularly those with more than seven digits. This is where the DNS comes to the rescue. A name server translates an IP address into a text or name address like this:

USM.MAINE.EDU

This represents a node, which is a specific computer. Like your street address, each part has a specific meaning. From left to right, the address goes from specific to general, just like your street address goes from top to bottom, specific to general. A DNS address breaks down like this:

USM The name of the local computer; in this case, it is a server for the University of Southern Maine
MAINE A subdomain, here referring to the University of Maine
EDU The domain or type of institution

EDU refers to an educational institution. Other domains you may see include GOV for government, MIL for military, COM for commercial organizations, ORG for other organizations, and NET for network resources. Note that these extensions refer to addresses from the US. For Internet travel outside of the US, there are sets of two letter domains, which correspond to the highest level domains for countries. For example, CA is Canada, UK is the United Kingdom, and ZA is South Africa. The United States has a country code (US) which is usually preceded by the state code (i.e., ME.US for Maine). In the US, most computers use the organizational domain names rather than the geographical name. Note that the two are not interchangeable. Using the example from above,

USM.MAINE.EDU

is not the same address as:

USM.ME.US.

If you tried to send mail to the latter, it would be returned with a message: "unknown host address."
All Internet addresses, regardless of the interface used, are based on the DNS.
An e-mail address has two parts: a user identification (user ID) and a node, joined together by the @ sign. An address can look as simple as:

LeslieN@USM.MAINE.EDU

where the User ID is LeslieN and the node is USM.MAINE.EDU (which is one of the nodes for the University of Southern Maine). Sometimes an address can be filled with odd symbols like !% or similar characters designed to guide the message between various smaller local area networks.
As noted earlier, your ISP will determine your e-mail address. The one just given in this example is my e-mail address at the university; my home e-mail is LNICOLL@MAINE.RR.COM. Can you figure this one out? Use the same steps as before: LNICOLL is my user name; MAINE is a node of the Time Warner Road-Runner Service; RR refers to RoadRunner; and COM is commercial. RoadRunner users around the country have similar addresses, but the node changes to reflect their community; that is, USER@TAMPABAY.RR.COM is the service in Tampa, Florida.
The URL is the standardized addressing scheme for sites on the WWW. Bear in mind that URLs require the use of a Web browser. A typical URL looks like this:

http://www.nursingcenter.com/journals

(This happens to be the address of the WWW site for the journals section of NursingCenter. You can link to *Computers in Nursing* from this site.)

As with other Internet addresses, there is a method to what appears at first glance to be madness. It breaks down like this:

access_type://domain.name/directory_name/file.name

Using the NursingCenter URL mentioned earlier, the address is broken down as follows:

- http:// refers to HyperText Transfer Protocol. This is the "language" of the WWW. All URLs begin with this, but you don't need to type it in; it is automatically inserted when you type the rest of the URL.
- WWW refers to World Wide Web. Most URLs begin with WWW, but not all.
- Nursingcenter is the domain name for the site.
- /journals is the directory path to the home page for the journals section of NursingCenter. Just what is a home page? I'll cover that in Chapter 3.

Practice reading domain names and URLs to become familiar with the language of the Internet. When someone gives you his or her e-mail address, inspect it. What is the extension? If it is .EDU, then that person may work at an educational institution or perhaps is a student. AOL.COM is the domain name for America Online, a very popular ISP. Learning how to decipher the URL can be a great boon to you in your Internet exploring.

Learning the Language

The Internet world is full of glyphs, acronyms, and slang. The savvy traveler has an understanding of the language of the land. Although much of what is written on the Internet is in English, without some familiarity with the unique language of the Internet, you can quickly become confused as to what is really being said.

Display 2-2 is a glossary of common terms and acronyms. Note that this is just a starting point. There are lots of dictionaries on the Internet, so if you come across a term that is not on my list, you might want to check an online glossary. http://www.computeruser.com/resources/dictionary/dictionary.html is one resource that I can recommend. Included in the list are common acronyms; again, this is just a sampling of some of the most common abbreviations that are frequently seen on the Internet. Abbreviations are very common. Because the majority of communications on the Internet are text based—that is, someone has to sit and type at a keyboard (even a graphic starts out as text)—it only makes sense that abbreviations have become popular. Why type out "frequently asked questions" when the acronym FAQ will do? If you come across an acronym that is not on my list, visit http://www.acronymfinder.com/ to find more than 137,000 acronyms and their meanings.

Acronyms have taken on a life of their own on the Internet. For nurses, these abbreviations often have dual meanings. PRN (pro re nata) means "as needed" to

DISPLAY 2-2. GLOSSARY OF COMMON INTERNET TERMS AND ACRONYMS

Address
The unique identifier for a specific location on a network. There are three types of addresses in common use within the Internet: e-mail addresses, IP or Internet address, and hardware or MAC addresses.

Application
Any of a class of "programs" or "software" that causes a computer to perform some useful function (like type text or add numbers or communicate over telephone lines).

Bandwidth
Technically, the difference, in Hertz (Hz), between the highest and lowest frequencies of a transmission channel. However, as typically used, the amount of data, usually measured in bits per second, that can be sent through a given communications circuit.

Banner
A popular type of advertising found on the WWW consisting of a graphic (usually banner shaped) that acts as a link to the advertiser's home page or other informational site.

BBS
Bulletin board system

Bookmark
A personal list of frequently accessed Web sites that you can create within your browser software.

BPS
Bits per second. The speed at which bits are transmitted over a communications system.

BRB
Bathroom break

Browser
An application that displays HTML and other information found on the Internet. Communicator, Internet Explorer, and Mosaic are examples of browsers. This client software accesses the World Wide Web and Gopher services, and lets you drift from link to link without having to have a purposeful search. Browsers encourage discovery by serendipity; hence, the name.

BTW
By the way

Client
A computer system or process that requests a service of another computer system or process (e.g., a computer requesting the contents of a file from a file server). In client-server computing, the client is the "front-end" program that the user runs to connect with, and request information from, the server program. For most of the common Internet tools, many different client programs are designed to work in DOS, Windows, Macintosh, and UNIX environments.

(continued)

DISPLAY 2-2. GLOSSARY OF COMMON INTERNET TERMS AND ACRONYMS (CONTINUED)

Client-server computing

The model or scheme underlying practically all programs running on the Internet (as well as other network and database software). In this design, the work of an application (such as FTP or Gopher) is divided up between two programs—the client (or "front end") and the server (or "back end"). The client program handles the work of connecting to the server and requesting files or information, and the server handles the work of finding and "serving up" the information (or of providing some other service, such as directing print jobs to a printer).

Congestion

What occurs when the load exceeds the capacity of a data communication path. You may be experiencing congestion when any of the following happens: you get a busy signal when you dial into a modem pool, the response from the server or host you are trying to reach is slow, or you get an error message telling you that no ports are available for the service or host you want to use.

Crash

An unexpected interruption of the proper functioning of a computer, disk drive, or software.

Cyberspace

Cyber comes from the '50s term "cybernetics," which is used to describe the science of computers. *Space* harkens to the '60s terms "inner space," "head space," and so on. *Cyberspace* is a term coined by either computer hackers or science fiction writers (both claim credit) to describe the place you are when you are traversing the virtual geography of the Internet. The term first appeared in print in William Gibson's novel *Neuromancer* (Ace, 1984) to describe the world of computers and the society that gathers around them.

Dial-up

A temporary, as opposed to dedicated, connection between computers established over a standard phone line.

Direct connection

Any Internet connection in which you have your own IP address and connect physically and directly to the Internet on a permanent basis via a dedicated phone line or network.

Directory

On a hard drive, a file which acts as a folder or drawer and contains other files or directories. On the Internet, a listing of Web sites, e-mail addresses, or other data.

Domain

A named collection of network hosts. Some important domains are: .com (commercial), .edu (educational), .net (network operations), .gov (US government), and .mil (US military). Most countries also have a domain. For example, .us (United States), .uk (United Kingdom), .au (Australia).

(continued)

DISPLAY 2-2. GLOSSARY OF COMMON INTERNET TERMS AND ACRONYMS (CONTINUED)

Domain Address or Domain Name System (DNS)
The human language name of a computer on the Internet, as opposed to its more computer-friendly numeric IP address. For example, hermes.merit.edu is a domain address and 42.1.1.6 is an IP address.

Domain Registration
The process of requesting and receiving a unique name for a location on the Internet from a regulatory body.

DSL
Digital subscriber line

E-mail (electronic mail)
A system whereby a computer user can exchange messages with other computer users (or groups of users) via a communications network. Electronic mail is one of the most popular uses of the Internet.

Emoticon
Common term for smiley face glyphs that are created with characters on the keyboard such as a colon, hyphen, and parenthesis :-).

Encryption
The manipulation of a packet's data in order to prevent any but the intended recipient from reading that data. There are many types of data encryption, which make up the basis of network security.

Ethernet
A local area network (LAN) transport protocol (TP), initially developed by Xerox and later refined by Digital, Intel, and Xerox IX. It is very common in computer networks. Its bandwidth is 10 megabit (10,000,000 bits per second). All hosts are connected to a coaxial cable, through which they contend for network access using a Carrier Sense Multiple Access with Collision Detection (CSMA/C paradigm).

FAQ
Frequently asked question (see below).

Firewall
A hardware device (or collection of devices) that is placed between two networks. One network is considered inside the company (safe) and one is considered outside the company (not safe). All traffic, both from the inside and outside, must pass through this device. The firewall limits access to authorized users and systems by filtering packets as they come in based on the source or destination address, as well as an application's TCP/IP port. On the Internet, firewall, bastion host, and secure Internet connection are synonymous.

(continued)

DISPLAY 2-2. GLOSSARY OF COMMON INTERNET TERMS AND ACRONYMS (CONTINUED)

Flame
A strong opinion or criticism of something, usually in a deliberately insulting tone, in an electronic mail message or news posting. Flames usually come in the form of grumpy, irritated, sometimes downright angry responses to questions or to inflammatory statements you make. Flaming is frowned upon in polite Internet society. It is common to precede a flame with an indication of pending fire (such as "FLAME ON!"). "Flame wars" occur when people start flaming other people for flaming when they shouldn't have. They can also start when a new reader in a newsgroup asks a question that older readers have answered many times and which has been incorporated into a FAQ. A warning to new users: some folks enjoy flame wars and deliberately try to provoke one. Sometimes, you'll be gang-flamed, in which case many (sometimes many, many, many) users will seek revenge on you (for whatever reason) by dumping your e-mail address with thousands upon thousands of worthless messages. Avoid flames. Be nice.

Forms-capable Browser
A World Wide Web browser that allows users to "fill in the blank" in questionnaires and other user-response items. Most GUI browsers are forms-capable, as are some of the line-mode browsers.

Frequently Asked Questions (FAQs)
A document containing answers to a set of such questions. Many newsgroups put out these FAQ documents so that each new person does not ask the same questions. Many computer product companies, as well as organizations that distribute information or do business over the Internet, have begun creating FAQs for their product, service, or information. Many FAQs are stored in an anonymous FTP archive, and many are broadcast across interested mailing lists at least once per month.

FTP
File transfer protocol. FTP is a method of sending files to and receiving files from a remote computer on the Internet. It is also the name of a program that uses the protocol to transfer files.

FYI
For your information

###
Grin; often used in e-mail and chats.

Gateway
The term "router" is now used in place of the original definition of "gateway." At present, a gateway is a communications device or program that passes data between networks having similar functions but dissimilar implementations. In other words, a gateway is a computer system that transfers data between normally incompatible applications or networks. It reformats the data so that they are acceptable for the new network (or application) before passing them on.

(continued)

Display 2-2. GLOSSARY OF COMMON INTERNET TERMS AND ACRONYMS (CONTINUED)

Glyph
The original term used by Fahlman to describe the smiley face created with a colon, hyphen, and parenthesis :-).

GUI
Graphical user interface. A GUI is a software "front end" that lets the user use pictures and "point-and-click" technology to access the software application. It allows a computer user to interact with the computer by manipulating graphic representations (icons) with a mouse or other pointing device instead of typing text commands. Many modern Internet clients are based on GUI principles and technology.

Header
The portion of a packet, preceding the actual data, containing source and destination addresses, and error checking and other fields. A header is also the part of an e-mail message that precedes the body of a message and contains, among other things, the message originator, date, and time.

Home Page
In the World Wide Web, a starting point for a set of information about a particular topic. In general terms, the home page is the default page that is presented when a user accesses a Web server.

Host
A computer that provides a physical link to the Internet and allows users to communicate with other host computers on a network. Individual users communicate by using application programs, such as electronic mail, telnet, and FTP. In some contexts, and in some philosophies of the way the Internet should work, the host itself is less important than the servers that run on it. For example, Web and Gopher servers distribute data to users without the user having to know which host the server is located on. A host computer is identified via its system and domain names. The terms "host," "site," and "server" all essentially are the same.

Hotlink
A word, phrase, graphic, or address that, when clicked on, loads other information about the linked phrase or loads a related Web page.

HTML
Hypertext markup language. Used to produce a hypertext document for display by a WWW browser; HTML uses a standardized set of tags that tells the browser how to display the text as well as how to specify hypertext links.

HTTP
Hypertext transfer protocol. A protocol that defines hypertext links to information on the WWW.

IAYF
Information at your fingertips. What many believe the Internet provides.

(continued)

Display 2-2. GLOSSARY OF COMMON INTERNET TERMS AND ACRONYMS (CONTINUED)

Icon
Graphic or symbol on the computer monitor that represents a computer task or file.

IMO; IMHO; IOHO
In my opinion; in my humble opinion; in our humble opinion

Internet service provider (ISP)
An Internet service provider charges start-up and monthly fees to users and provides them with the initial host connection to the rest of the Internet, usually via a dial-up connection.

IP
Internet protocol. It allows a packet of information to traverse multiple networks on the way to its final destination.

IP address
The 32-bit address defined by the Internet protocol that is usually represented in decimal notation. For example, an IP address looks like this: 127.0.0.1, whereas a domain name looks like this: nic.cicnet.net.

IRC
Internet relay chat. A worldwide "party line" protocol that allows users to converse with each other in real time. IRC is structured as a network of servers, each of which accepts connections from client programs, one per user. Some schools and organizations have disabled IRC on their computers and networks because of congestion problems or organizational policies about appropriate use. IRC garnered worldwide attention during the Gulf War, when citizens on their computers in Tel Aviv during the bombing raids were describing the events as they happened over IRC to listeners around the world.

Java
A platform-independent programming language developed by Sun Microsystems. Java applications are compiled and stored on a server and downloaded to be run on local "Java virtual machines" embedded into the client software.

Javascript
A special-purpose, Java-like language especially adept at interacting with user input and used extensively to make Web pages interactive.

JPEG
Joint photographic experts group, which defined a standard compression format for high-resolution color images.

LAN
Local area network

Load
In World Wide Web or Gopher sessions, a page or menu is loaded into your browser when you access that page and the images and text appear on your screen. If for some reason you need to update the image or information, you can reload the page or menu.

(continued)

Display 2-2. GLOSSARY OF COMMON INTERNET TERMS AND ACRONYMS (CONTINUED)

LOL

Laughing out loud

Lurking

On a mailing list or Usenet newsgroup, listening without responding publicly. As the name implies, this activity is considered somewhat antisocial, but lurking allows beginners to get a feel for the flavor and response patterns of the participants of the group and also lets them get up to speed on the history of the group.

Mailer

A program used to read and write electronic mail, such as Eudora or Pegasus.

MIME

Multipurpose Internet mail extensions. An extension to Internet e-mail that provides the ability to transfer nontextual data, such as graphics, audio, and faxes.

Netiquette

A pun on "etiquette" referring to proper behavior on a network. There is no "Miss Manners" of the Internet.

POP

1. Point of presence: a site where there exists a collection of telecommunications equipment, usually digital leased lines and multi-protocol routers, to physically connect users to the Internet. Many network providers have their equipment located along with telephone company POPs. 2. Post office protocol: a protocol designed to allow single-user hosts to read mail from a server. There are three versions: POP, POP2, and POP3. Later versions are not compatible with earlier versions.

POTS

Plain old telephone service. What modems use to connect to the Internet.

Port

Although your computer has a physical port in the back into which you plug things, TCP/IP ports are also values defined in the protocol. For example, most computers that accept Telnet sessions create a port "23" to accept Telnet transmissions. When a packet comes in with the Telnet request, it carries a request for port 23. Each application has a unique port number associated with it.

PPP

Point-to-point protocol. IETF (Internet Engineering Task Force) standard that provides a method for transmitting packets over serial point-to-point links. PPP is the successor protocol to SLIP and like SLIP allows dial-up users to connect their home computers to the Internet as peer hosts. Like SLIP, PPP establishes the initial connection between your computer and your service provider's host system, but includes a more robust set of protocols than SLIP. PPP is more efficient than SLIP when using a high-speed modem (14.4 kbps or higher). PPP can also be more difficult to configure than SLIP.

(continued)

Display 2-2. GLOSSARY OF COMMON INTERNET TERMS AND ACRONYMS (CONTINUED)

Protocol

A formal description of message formats and the rules two or more computers must follow to exchange those messages. Protocols can describe low-level details of computer-to-computer interfaces (for example, the order in which the bits from a byte are sent across a wire), or high-level exchanges between application programs (for example, the way in which two programs transfer a file across the Internet).

RFC

Request for comments

ROFL

Rolling on the floor, laughing

RSI

Repetitive strain injury. Not technically a computer abbreviation, but it shows up quite a bit in discussion groups.

RTM

Read the manual. Often an "F" is inserted between the "T" and the "M." I will leave that abbreviation to the reader's imagination.

Search Engine

A search engine is a computer program or group of programs that can take a search string (usually a word or words) and rapidly compare that string with the information in its database, keyword index, or the text of many documents.

Secure Server

A server, sometimes called a Secure Commerce Server, that encrypts the transfer of data to and from a user to protect his or her identity or sensitive data, such as credit card numbers, that may otherwise be intercepted.

Server

In client-server computing, the "back-end" program from which a client program requests information or other resources. The server handles the work of locating and extracting the information. The term is also often used to refer to the computer running a server program, particularly if it is used only for that purpose (as, for example, a "print server" in a LAN). Essentially means the same as host; however, the term "server" has come to take on a separate connotation, in which "server" is preceded by an adjective that identifies the type of Internet service it provides. For instance, you can connect to a Web server, an FTP server, a Gopher server, or a host (pun intended) of other server types.

Signature

The three- or four-line message at the bottom of an e-mail message that identifies the sender. Large signatures (over five lines) are generally frowned on. These files usually have the file name sig or signature. With many e-mail clients, this file is automatically appended to the sender's messages.

(continued)

**DISPLAY 2-2. GLOSSARY OF COMMON INTERNET
TERMS AND ACRONYMS (CONTINUED)**

SLIP
Serial line Internet protocol. A protocol used to run IP over serial lines, such as telephone circuits or RS-232 cables, interconnecting two systems. SLIP, along with PPP, is one of two popular protocols that allow home computer users to connect their computers to the Internet as peer hosts. SLIP and PPP encapsulate TCP/IP packets for transmission over phone lines.

SMTP
Simple mail transfer protocol. A protocol used to transfer electronic mail between computers. It is a server-to-server protocol, so other protocols are used to access the messages.

TCP/IP
Transmission control protocol over Internet protocol. A common shorthand that refers to the suite of transport and application protocols that runs over the Internet. TCP/IP is the set of rules that defines the communications standards for passing information back and forth across the Internet. TCP/IP is actually a collection of more than 100 transmission protocols. It is the common language that controls all communications hardware linked to the Internet, thereby helping to avoid communications conflicts and misunderstandings when data is shuttled among computers linked to the Internet.

TIFF
Tagged Interchange File Format, a graphics format mutually established by Adobe and Microsoft for use in importing graphics into different applications. TIFF is a common graphics standard among PC applications, but it cannot be used with some GIF/JPEG viewers.

URL
Universal resource locator. A standard for specifying the address of a document on the Internet, such as a home page, a file, or a newsgroup.

Viewer
A software utility that allows you to open and view any of a variety of file formats (typically GIF and JPEG) images online.

WWW
World Wide Web

Zip
A compression format used to make files smaller, often before sending them over the Internet. A decompression program such as WinZip is needed to make these files usable after downloading.

a nurse but means "printer" in the computer world. Other examples are OS (left eye [nursing], operating system [computer]), and CAD (coronary artery disease [nursing], computer-aided design [computer]). Teeter and Wellman[1] have written an amusing article with more examples of similar acronyms in nursing and computer terms; when you read it, it will be clear why you should not trust your nursing judgment to translate Internet acronyms!

Smiley face glyphs, also called *emoticons*, are very popular and are illustrated in Figure 2-1. Scott Fahlman, a research computer scientist at Carnegie Mellon

The following list of emoticons has been accumulated over the years. Enjoy!

Full Version		Abbreviated Version
:-)	Happy	:)
(-:	Left handed/Australian	(:
:-(	Sad	:(
;-)	Winky/tongue-in-cheek	;)
#-)	Oh, what a night!	#)
:-O	Yelling/shocked	:O
:-I	Frowning	:I

For those wanting a more "aesthetically pleasing" emoticon you can use the profile version … some examples are below:

:^) :^] ;^)

So, when words absolutely fail you …

~~:-[	Net flame	8-)	Wears glasses
:-$	Put your money where your mouth is	B:-)	Wears sunglasses on head
:-P	Sticking out tongue	:-T	Keeping a straight face/tight-lipped
:-@	Screaming/swearing/very angry/about to be sick	:-y	Said with a smile
:*)	Drunk/clown	:-I	Disgusted/grim/no expression
>;->	Wicked grin	:~-(	Crying/shed a tear
:-#	Been smacked In the mouth/wears a brace/kiss	:'-(	Crying
R-)	Broken glasses	:~(~~	Crying
(:-)	Bald	:-Q	A smoker
:-)))	Is very fat	:-?	A smoker
:-{}	Wears lipstick	I-o	Bored
@:-)	Wears a turban	:-X	A kiss/lips are sealed
>;->	Leering	(:-D	Has a big mouth
$-)	Yuppie/just won a large sum of money	(:+)	Has a big nose
:'(	Crying	:-{{	Has a moustache
:=)	Two noses	:-*	Just ate something sour/bitter taste/kiss
8:]	Gorilla	[:-)	Is wearing a walkman

FIGURE 2-1. Popular emoticons.

University (CMU), first suggested these little glyphs. In describing his idea, Fahlman writes, "I am the one who first suggested the use of the :-) and :-(glyphs in E-mail and bulletin board posts sometime around 1981. People were making sarcastic comments in posts, and others were taking them more seriously than they were intended (no body language on the net), and silly arguments were breaking out. So I suggested on one of the CMU bulletin boards that people explicitly label comments not meant to be serious with a :-) glyph. Very quickly this idea spread all around the world, and others started creating clever variations on the theme. The awful term 'emoticons' is much more recent."[2]

To see how a glyph such as this works, turn your head sideways. Be forewarned: some people cannot stand glyphs; others sprinkle them liberally through all their messages. You'll soon develop your own style and will learn what is acceptable within your circle of e-mail colleagues.

REFERENCES

1. Teeter M, Wellman D. When is DOS not DOS? *Computers in Nursing* 1995;13(6):301–302.
2. E-mail message from Scott Fahlman to Don E. Z'Boray, available online at http://www.Newbie.net/JumpStations/SmileyFAQ/Fahlman.html

CHAPTER 3

■■

Site-Seeing Tips for the Internet Traveler

MODES OF TRAVEL DURING YOUR INTERNET JOURNEY

The Internet is a network of networks all working together to form a global community. The Internet uses unique addresses that can be used to locate information and specialized software to let you virtually visit faraway places and move information around the world. Just as you need to decide whether to take a bus, drive a car, or ride a train on a traditional trip, you need to determine what mode of travel is appropriate on your Internet exploration. Different sites require different methods of transportation. This chapter is an introduction to different ways of travel and unique sites you can expect to see during your Internet journey.

Some people think that the Internet is a fairly recent development. Actually, the Internet has been around for more than 3 decades. It started out as a U.S. Defense Department network called the *ARPAnet* in 1969. Since then, it has grown, changed, matured, and mutated, but the essential structure of interconnected domains randomly distributed throughout the world has remained the same. As a matter of fact, ARPAnet no longer exists, but many of the standards established for that first network still govern the communication and structure of the modern Internet.

An important feature of the Internet, which has been constant since the beginning, is the notion of widely distributed, interconnected computers forming a vast network. In other words, there is not a huge, central computer somewhere that all information passes through. Rather, there are millions of interconnected computers forming a vast, worldwide network. Remember that the original Internet came from military roots: if there was one large computer, that computer could be located and destroyed. By having the system be based on a network of individual computers, the entire network became more stable in the event of nuclear attack.

Many of the popular features of the Internet have come from these same military roots. E-mail was developed to provide a method of communication in the event that the telephone system was destroyed. Global positioning satellites were developed to provide tracking and locating of planes and missiles. Virtual reality was used to train pilots to fly in horrific conditions. Today, we continue to benefit from many of these developments that were created in anticipation of a nuclear war, which thankfully did not come to pass. But because ARPAnet was first and foremost a military application, the early development of the Internet was shrouded in secrecy, which some contend impeded its development.

Consequently, for many years, the Internet was more or less the private domain of scientists, researchers, and university professors who used the Internet to communicate and to exchange files and software. A number of events transpired in the 1980s and early 1990s that opened up the Internet, resulting in its enormous growth and ensuing popularity. Some of the changes were political, such as the High-Performance Computing Act of 1991, sponsored by then-Senator Al Gore; some were logistical, such as the decision to allow computers other than those used for research and military purposes to connect to the network; and some were just plain practical, such as the development of so-called user-friendly software and tools that allowed less-experienced computer users to obtain information easily and quickly.

As noted earlier, the first uses of the Internet were primarily communication and sharing of information. The tools used to accomplish these tasks were e-mail (for communication) and remote login, which had two functions: telnet (for browsing another computer) and file transfer protocol (FTP; for transferring files between computers). The original versions of the software for these tasks grew from either mainframe computer roots or Unix workstations. (Unix is a popular operating system that was developed at the University of California at Berkeley.) In recent years, a variety of software programs, such as Pegasus Mail or Eudora (for e-mail) and Gopher, Communicator, and Internet Explorer (for browsing and sharing files) have all been developed. At their hearts, these programs are designed for the same original Internet activities of communication and information sharing, but they make the process much easier, allowing the more novice or casual computer user access to the same resources that the experts enjoyed for many years.

Internet travel is still based on e-mail and remote login, with its activities of telnet and FTP. When you use a program such as Communicator on the WWW, you may not realize that you are remotely connecting to another computer or using FTP to download files, but you are. It is possible to travel the Internet without knowing anything about how the system works, but I have found that if you have even a brief understanding of these tools, your trip is more likely to be successful. How you get around governs the sites and information that are available to you. Having an understanding of how you are getting around allows you to more efficiently find the type of information you are seeking.

COMMUNICATION: ELECTRONIC MAIL

Individual E-Mail

By far, the most common use of the Internet is to send *electronic mail* (e-mail). It is also very easy. Exchanging e-mail with colleagues is probably the best way to become comfortable with the electronic world. Sending electronic mail across international networks is almost as easy as sending paper mail, but it arrives in seconds or minutes, rather than days.

To send e-mail you need three things: Internet access and an e-mail address (this was discussed in Chapter 2), someone to send mail to, and a mail program. I am assuming you have made an Internet connection and have your own personal e-mail address. At the time you set that up, you should also have gotten a mail program, either one that is part of your browser or a stand-alone program. So the last step is finding someone to send your first message to: if all else fails, send one to me at LeslieN@usm.maine.edu!

How can you find other e-mail addresses? The easiest and most reliable method is to ask someone for his or her address. Write it down, and after you send a message to the person in question, store the address in the address book contained in the mail program. E-mail addresses are finicky: a misspelling will cause the mail to be returned to you (or worse, your private message will go to the wrong person!). I speak from experience. My name has several "L"s that people often mistake for the number 1 or the letter "e." Another common mistake that people make is to leave the "e" off of the word "Maine." Each of these very simple (and obvious) errors will mean that your message does not get to me. Once you have a person's correct e-mail address, which you have used to send a message successfully, store it in your address book. That way, you'll never have to type the address again. Figure 3-1 is an illustration of the address book feature in Pegasus Mail.

There are other ways to obtain e-mail addresses. With the popularity of the Internet, many people include their e-mail on their business cards. I suggest that you do the same. It is also possible to search for people on the Internet. A number of programs, such as Switchboard (www.switchboard.com) and WhoWhere? (www.whowhere.com) have been developed for the express purpose of locating names, addresses, and e-mail addresses of people throughout the world. I'll be honest: in my experience, "people search engines" such as these are not terribly reliable, but they are certainly worth a try and a good starting point to find an old friend or colleague. If you know where someone works, that may be another way to do a successful people search. Universities tend to have comprehensive faculty lists that include e-mail addresses; professional associations, such as the Association of periOperative Registered Nurses (AORN), also include staff directories. With a minimum level of resourcefulness, you should be able to locate electronically connected long-lost friends and relatives by using the Internet.

E-mail tends to be informal, and most recipients are tolerant of "less-than-perfect" communications. Even so, if your mail program includes features such as

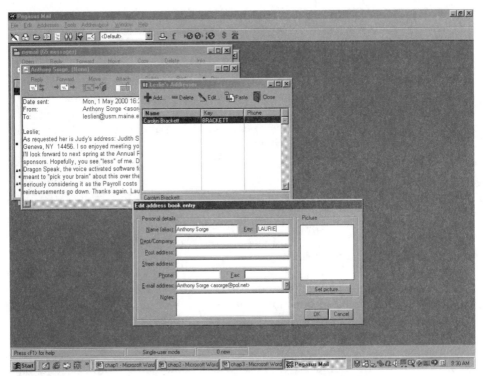

FIGURE 3-1. Illustration of the address book feature in Pegasus Mail.

a spell-checker, I suggest you use it. Another useful feature is to create a signature file. With a signature file, certain information, such as your name, e-mail address, and phone number, will be appended to every message you send. My signature file includes my name, title, university address, phone number, fax number, and e-mail address. Having the signature file saves me several hundred keystrokes a day and also ensures that those receiving my message know how to get in touch with me. Some people include inspirational quotes or lines of poetry in their signatures. These can be fun, but don't get too carried away: this is a signature, not an epitaph!

A few words of warning about e-mail. One: TYPING IN ALL CAPITALS IS NOT A GOOD IDEA. In popular *netiquette* (etiquette for the Internet) terms, typing exclusively in capital letters is considered shouting and very rude. Turn the caps lock off before you send your message.

Two: just because e-mail is simple and informal, don't forget rules of common courtesy. If you are writing to someone you don't know to request information, include a brief introduction. Who are you and why do you need this information? This sounds obvious, but I get messages with no introduction and no signature that say things like: "Pls help. I'm doing a paper on computers. Send me articles about computers and nsg thx." You can be sure these types of messages go instantly into the trash bin.

Three: be careful with attachments. Attachments are appended to e-mail messages and contain files or pictures. Although attachments are very useful for transmitting information to others, it is also possible to send a virus to someone else via an attachment. I have a standing policy of accepting attachments only from people I know or from people who have forewarned me that they are going to be sending me something via an attachment. Anonymous attachments go right into the trash bin.

Another problem is spam: junk e-mail. Junk e-mail can fill up your electronic mailbox just as quickly as traditional junk fills your home mailbox. There are many different types of spam: messages selling goods and services, get-rich-quick schemes, chain letters, and hoaxes. My advice for the best approach for all of these types of spam is simple: HIT THE DELETE KEY. This is the easiest and simplest solution, but too often people don't take this advice.

Many of the spam messages you receive may include a line such as, "If you do not wish to receive further messages of this type, send a reply and request to be removed from the mailing list." Trust me, that is the worst thing you can do! By replying to the message, you confirm your e-mail address. Instead of removing your name from the list, you run the risk of exponentially increasing the spam e-mail that you receive.

If spam is a real problem for you, consider contacting your ISP to determine whether they can filter the messages in question. You are paying for a service from your ISP and should reasonably expect that they can (and will) stop annoying messages selling laser toner or XXX-rated pictures. If your ISP cannot provide this service, you might consider changing your ISP.

E-mail chain letters and hoaxes are another problem. It is amazing to me how many people will temporarily suspend all rational thinking to forward a chain letter to hundreds of their friends and colleagues, with the misguided belief that such forwarding is actually going to make a difference. But this is simply not the case. The American Cancer Society (ACS) and the Make-A-Wish Foundation have both been targets of e-mail chain letters that purport to do good, but have cost both organizations money and valuable human resources to deal with the problems. The ACS has a notice on its Website that reads:

"The American Cancer Society is greatly disturbed by reports of a fraudulent chain letter circulating on the internet which lists the American Cancer Society as a 'corporate sponsor' but which has in no way been endorsed by the American Cancer Society. There are several variations of this letter in circulation. . . If you want to help fight cancer, please consider giving a donation or joining a local community event like Relay For Life."

The site also lists Websites that you can go to to debunk hoaxes and chain letters, including

- urbanlegends.about.com (one of my favorites);
- kumite.com/myths/;
- nonprofit.net/hoax/hoax.html; and
- hoaxkill.com/index2.html

If you receive an e-mail chain letter, hoax, or virus alert, read it (if you wish) and then delete it. Do not forward it to friends, relatives, and colleagues as the letter suggests. If, for some reason, you believe this message is legitimate, then I suggest you go to the one of the aforementioned sites (the Urban Legend site at about.com is very comprehensive) and determine whether you can find more information about the letter, hoax, or virus. In all likelihood, you will and probably get a good laugh in the process. If, on the other hand, you do not find the information you are looking for, that still does not mean you should forward the message to others. Particularly in the case of virus alerts, go to your ISP, or if you are at work, to someone in your IS or computer services department. Let that person do the necessary research and take necessary action if he or she determines that this is a real problem.

Group E-Mail: Mailing Lists

A very popular feature of the Internet is *mailing lists*, which provide a forum for groups of people with similar interests to get together and share their information through a mail-based discussion group. These lists can range in size from a few dozen people to thousands, and they can generate anywhere from a few messages a week to a hundred or more in a day. There are hundreds of thousands of mailing lists, on topics ranging from arts, cars, conspiracy theories, hobbies, favorite authors, and yes, even nursing! Being on a mailing list can put information and resources literally at your fingertips. Imagine asking 900 of your colleagues around the world a question concerning a clinical problem and receiving an answer within minutes, or discussing US healthcare reform with health workers from other nations.

Some have called lists an acquired taste. Personally, I enjoy lists and I subscribe to several, both for nursing as well as personal interests. My husband, on the other hand, cannot stand mailing lists. He doesn't like dealing with the volume of messages, and he gets tired of the sometimes inane conversations. If you have never been on a mailing list, I suggest you try subscribing and see what you think. If it is not your cup of tea, it is easy enough to unsubscribe, as you will learn in the following discussion.

MECHANICS OF MAILING LISTS

All Internet mailing lists work in a similar fashion. As noted earlier, each list is developed around a particular topic or interest area. If you are interested in this topic, you may choose to subscribe to the list. Unlike subscribing to a magazine, there is no charge to subscribe to an Internet mailing list. Once you are subscribed, you can send messages to the list. You will also receive messages from the list, which you can read, reply to, or delete. The communications are *asynchronous*; that is, the discussions are not occurring in real time, such as you would have during a conversation. Instead, the discussions occur via e-mail, with one person asking a question or posing a comment, and then other members of the list replying.

Even though the discussions are not synchronous, they are real discussions with sometimes heated debates!

A mailing list is run from a computer, often a mainframe, that has the software necessary to automatically manage the list (subscribing members, sending messages, and so on). There are five major software programs that manage mailing lists: LISTSERV, LISTPROC, MAILSERV, MAILBASE, and MAJORDOMO. Although these programs are similar, they each have their own little quirks. For example, four of the five programs use the word "Subscribe" to subscribe to a list, whereas MAILBASE uses the word "Join." As a user, you don't need to worry too much about the software, but you should be aware that there are different programs managing the mailing lists. You can usually figure out which software a system is using by inspecting the address of the list. For example, the NURSENET list is on a system using LISTSERV software (LISTSERV@LISTSERV. UTORONTO.CA). NURSE-ROGERS is on a system using MAILBASE (MAIL- BASE@ MAILBASE.AC.UK); NPINFO is MAJORDOMO (Majordomo@nurse.net); PERIOP is LISTPROC (LISTPROC@U.WASHINGTON.EDU) and PEDIATRIC- PAIN is MAILSERV (MAILSERV@AC.DAL.CA). Descriptions of all of these lists are included in the directory; a summary of the different mail server commands for the different programs can be found in Display 3-1.

Generally, mailing list discussion groups can be divided into two types: layperson oriented and professional oriented. The person who originally created the list, known as the list owner, will set the tone and the direction of the list; if the discussions get too far off track, the list owner may intervene to get the conversation back on topic.

How do you find out what mailing lists exist? Many of the popular nursing lists are listed in the "Directory of Sites" in Part II. Websites on certain topics often have links to mailing lists on the same topic. You can also visit Liszt (www.liszt.com), which is a "list of lists" with over 87,000 entries. Finally, ask friends and colleagues. If you have electronically connected friends with similar interests, they may already be subscribing to a list that would interest you.

To join a mailing list, you subscribe by sending an e-mail message to the computer that is hosting the list. The format for subscribing is pretty standard from list to list. As an example, to subscribe to NURSERES, a discussion group concerning nursing research and related issues, you would send a message to LISTSERV@KENTVM.KENT.EDU. Leave the "from" and "subject" lines blank. Note that when you do this, your mail program may ask you if you intended to send the message with a blank subject line—answer "yes." In the first line of the message, type: subscribe NURSERES <your name>; insert your name, such as Jane Doe, as you want it to appear on the subscription list. If you have an automatic signature added to your mail messages, turn that feature off before you send a subscription request. Figure 3-2 is an example of a completed subscription message. Once the message is received, one of the following will happen:

- Your message is rejected, which usually means you made a mistake. Go back and carefully check your message; make sure that the subject line is blank

Display 3-1. BASIC COMMANDS FOR COMMON MAILING LIST SOFTWARE

Note: Commands such as "subscribe," "unsubscribe," or "review" are sent directly to the list server. Usually that address begins "listserv," "majordomo," or "listname-request" @domain-name. Some basic commands and the syntax required by different software systems are shown below.

Messages for distribution to the subscribers must be sent to an entirely different address. Usually that address begins "listname" @domainname.

When you subscribe to a discussion group it will automatically send you basic information about the group, including how to post messages and how to unsubscribe. It is a good idea to save that message.

Important note: Many mailing lists are very particular about the address you use for sending commands or posting messages. Be sure to subscribe to a discussion group from the same e-mail address you plan to use for receiving and posting messages or your messages may be refused. You should unsubscribe and then resubscribe when you change e-mail addresses.

A. Listserv Discussion Groups (most common type for university-based lists)

Subscribe: subscribe [listname] {firstname lastname}
Unsubscribe: unsubscribe [listname] or signoff [listname]
Receive digest version: set [listname] digest
Vacation, stop mail: set [listname] nomail
Resume mail: set [listname] mail or set [listname] digest
Get list of subscribers: review [listname]
Receive a copy of your posts: set [listname] repro
Receive acknowledgment of your posts: set [listname] ack

Example of a Listserv discussion group: NURSENET

B. Majordomo Discussion Groups

Subscribe: subscribe [listname] [e-mail-address]
Unsubscribe: unsubscribe [listname]
Digest: subscribe [listname]-digest
Cancel digest: unsubscribe [listname]-digest
List of subscribers: who [listname]
(A copy of your post is sent automatically; no option for vacation/no mail)

Example of a Majordomo discussion group: NPINFO

C. Listproc Discussion Groups

Subscribe: subscribe [listname] {firstname lastname}
Unsubscribe: unsubscribe [listname] {firstname lastname}
Vacation stop: set [listname] mail postpone

(continued)

Display 3-1. BASIC COMMANDS FOR
COMMON MAILING LIST SOFTWARE (CONTINUED)

Resume delivery: set [listname] mail ack
Digest: set [listname] mail digest
Cancel digest: set [listname] mail ack
List of subscribers: recipients [listname]
Copy of your posts: set [listname] mail ack

Example of a Listproc discussion group: PERIOP

D. Mailbase Discussion Groups (Mailbase is a popular program in the UK)

Subscribe: join [list] {firstname lastname}
Unsubscribe: leave [list] {firstname lastname}
Vacation stop: suspend mail [listname]
Resume delivery: resume mail [listname]
List of subscribers: review [listname]
Copy of your posts: standard feature; you always receive your own messages
Digest: not supported

Example of a Mailbase discussion group: NURSE-ROGERS

E. Mailserv Discussion Groups

Subscribe: subscribe [listname] {firstname lastname}
Unsubscribe: unsubscribe [listname] {firstname lastname}
List of subscribers: send/list [listname]
Copy of your posts: standard feature; you always receive your own messages
Vacation stop, Digest: not supported

Example of a Mailserv discussion group: PEDIATRIC-PAIN

and that you correctly typed the address of the list (it is common for people to put an "e" at the end of LISTSERV, which will cause your message to be rejected). Once you recheck your message and correct any mistakes, try sending it again.

- You will automatically be added to the list, in which case you will receive a message confirming your registration and welcoming you to the group.
- You will be requested to send a confirmation; once the confirmation is received, you will be sent a welcome.
- Your name will be forwarded to the list owner for processing. Based on the decision of the list owner, you will (or will not) be added to the group.

High-volume lists usually ask for a confirmation message to be sent. This protects you from being subscribed to a list without your knowledge. It is becoming

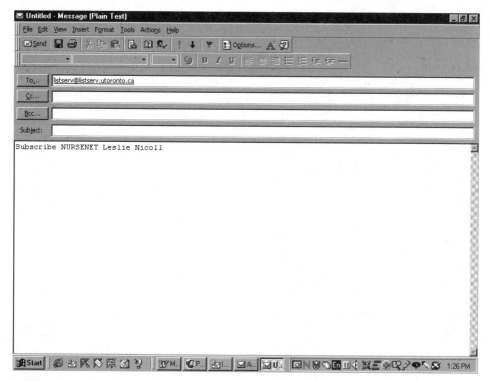

FIGURE 3-2. Subscription to NURSENET e-mail message.

the most common response to your request to subscribe. The confirmation message that you receive (see an example in Figure 3-3) will give instructions on how to reply to the message and confirm your subscription. Once that is done, you will receive a welcome message and be part of the list.

Private or confidential lists often require screening. For example, AANURSES is a mailing list for nurses and other healthcare professionals in recovery from alcohol and substance abuse. Because of the nature of the discussion, and the goal of the list members to create a safe environment for its members, a person desiring to subscribe to the list must write to the list owner and describe the reason for wishing to join. Another wrinkle, just to keep you on your toes: this particular list has a slightly different method for subscribing. You send a message to AANURSES@ONTONSYSTEMS.COM. Put the word "subscribe" (no quotes) in the SUBJECT field. Leave the message blank. The list owner will contact you privately to confirm your subscription.

Once your subscription is successfully processed, you'll get an automatically generated message informing you that you are subscribed. You'll often get a message from the list owner, welcoming you to the group and informing you about list netiquette. The welcome message usually includes helpful information on

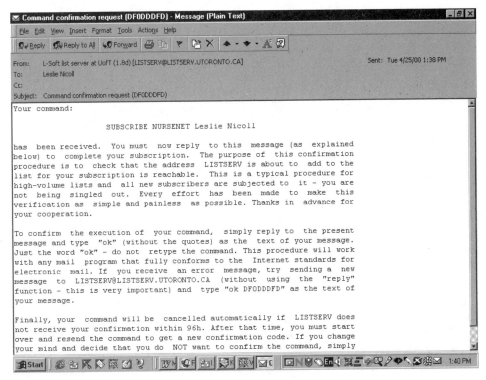

FIGURE 3-3. Confirmation request for the NURSENET mailing list.

how to *unsubscribe,* or stop the mail. It is a good idea to print the message and save it for future reference.

Once you are a member of a mailing list, messages can be sent to all of the subscribers by addressing the message to the list. For the nursing research list, the address is NURSERES@KENTVM.KENT.EDU. Note how the name of the list is now in the address, where before it was the name of the software. Be forewarned, some active lists may generate 20, 30, or more messages a day. If you are paying for a connection that charges for messages received, it could get expensive. If your mailbox is small, messages will bounce back to the list owner or the list, which is also a source of aggravation for the members.

Digest is a feature that can help you manage the volume of mail. When you receive a list in digest form, the messages are bundled and sent in one large group. Messages are bundled when they reach a total of 500 lines, which typically is between 10 and 15 messages. So instead of receiving 50 messages in a day, you might receive 3 or 4. Keep in mind that you are still getting all the messages, they just come in large groups instead of individually.

All lists have owners but that does not mean the list is moderated. In a *moderated discussion*, all messages go to the list owner before they are posted to the list.

In an *unmoderated discussion*, the messages automatically go to the entire list. There are advantages and disadvantages to each. In a moderated list, all the error messages (the ones that say "How do I unsubscribe from this list?" over and over) will be deleted. Similarly, wildly inappropriate messages never make it to the group. On the other hand, some people find the moderating process to be uncomfortably akin to censorship. Which is better? You can decide after you experience both types of lists. Of the lists mentioned previously, NURSERES is moderated but NURSENET is not.

Closed lists also exist. A *closed list* is one in which the subscribers are restricted; for example, students registered in a particular class may be the only people able to subscribe to a list. Generally, the addresses of closed lists are not made public, but it is possible to search on a mainframe to find out the names of all lists that reside on that mainframe. If you try to subscribe to a list and your subscription is refused, it may be because it is a closed list. A closed list is similar to a private or confidential list mentioned earlier.

Mailing List Etiquette

Mailing lists have their own personalities, and certain rules of etiquette govern your participation. When you first subscribe to a list, you might choose to "lurk" for awhile to get a sense of the list. By reading the messages and seeing the types of responses, you will get a feel for the members of the community. Once you decide to post a message to the list, an introduction is usually in order. This doesn't have to be lengthy or terribly detailed, but a short, "Hi, my name is. . . , I work in. . . , My interests are. . ." message is usually appreciated by the group.

Many lists have archives of "frequently asked questions" (FAQs) that you might want to consult. It can be very frustrating to list members to have a newcomer dive in with a question that has been asked many times before and for which an answer is available online in the archive.

When you post a question, be clear and to the point. Tell people what information you want and how you want it. Do you want everyone to post their replies to the list or to send you responses privately? Similarly, if you are replying to a message, note to whom you are replying. By default, all responses go to the whole list. If you want to reply to the original poster privately, make sure to double-check that you have the correct e-mail address in the address line.

Cut and paste when you reply to a message. That helps others remember the content of the original message, but by editing it, everyone does not have to read the entire message again. Remember, mailing lists are discussions, so do your part to keep the discussion focused and on track. Cut and paste is especially important if you receive the list in a digest version; if you press reply and don't edit the message, the whole digest (all 500 lines of messages) will go back to the entire list.

If the nature of the topic changes, change the subject line. This allows the list members to quickly scan and delete the messages that are not of interest.

Flaming is not a good idea. A *flame* is when someone attacks another person, usually in a virulent and violent manner. Remember that the whole point of a list is to have a discussion; it is possible to disagree with someone's ideas, but that does not mean you have to denigrate the person in the process. In my experience, nurses on mailing lists are generally very supportive and treat each other respectfully. But there are flame-throwers out there, so forewarned is forearmed.

Do not send attachments to the list. Remember that a list may have many hundreds of subscribers, some of whom may be running very plain vanilla computer systems that cannot handle sophisticated graphics or large files. Others may be paying by the minute for their Internet connection; large files, such as those found in attachments, are not going to be seen favorably. Finally, viruses are usually transmitted in attachments, so you run the risk of infecting the entire list if you send an attachment that contains a virus. All of these are valid reasons for why you should not send attachments to a list.

Keep in mind how mailing lists work: you send administrative messages (subscribe, unsubscribe, and so on) to the mainframe, usually to the "listserv@listserv"-type address. Messages to the list go to "listname@listserv." All of us have made the mistake of sending an administrative message to the list, but doing that too often is sure to guarantee that you will make someone very angry, and you will probably get flamed as a result.

Newbies (newcomers) are afforded a wide degree of latitude and mistakes are expected and accepted, but do your best to learn the ropes and manage your subscription in a responsible and professional manner. Although list owners are loathe to do this, they can involuntarily unsubscribe those people who repeatedly post off topic, flame others, send viruses, or mismanage their account. Keep all of these points in mind when you join a list.

Electronic Publications

A close cousin of Listserv groups are electronic publications. Although they do not invite discussion, most are subscribed to and distributed in the same manner as the discussion groups. Many electronic publications are distributed free to subscribers across the Internet. They vary in frequency, but all offer timely information to the health and medical community and most welcome reader interaction. Figure 3-4 is an illustration of an electronic newsletter distributed by the Agency for Healthcare Research and Quality (AHRQ).

Usenet News Groups

Usenet news groups are topical discussion special interest groups, similar in many ways to mailing list discussion groups. Unlike lists, in which one has to subscribe to receive messages by e-mail, the posts in the Usenet groups are stored on the mainframe computer for a period of time. Think of the difference between receiving mail and reading a bulletin board. With a mailing list, you get the mail in your mailbox and have to deal with it, even if that means simply hitting the delete key. With Usenet groups, you are reading the messages posted on a bulletin board. If you do not happen to walk by the bulletin board, you will not see the messages.

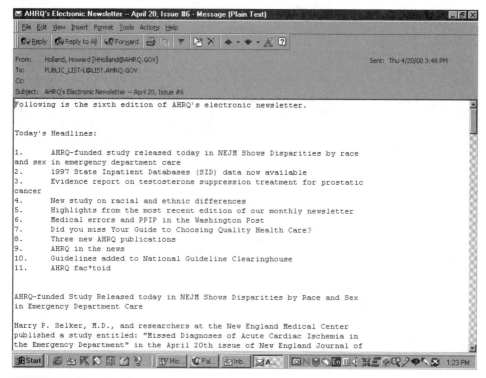

FIGURE 3-4. Example of an electronic newsletter.

As a point of information, some mailing list discussions are also echoed to the news groups. This gives you the opportunity to choose how you get your information. For example, the Listserv STAT-L is a consultation group for statistics. It is echoed to the Usenet group sci.stat.consult. If you are a researcher who is engaged in statistical analysis on a regular basis, you might appreciate the ongoing discussion of statistical procedures, problems, and solutions. On the other hand, if you are a more casual user, you might be glad to know about the sci.stat.consult group but choose to read it only when you have a specific question in mind that you would like to have answered.

Just about every topic imaginable is covered somewhere in a Usenet news group. Just as mailing lists are an acquired taste, so are the news groups. It is common to hear people refer to the "signal-to-noise" ratio in the newsgroups: for the 1 bit of useful information, there are 99 bits of junk. Some people get tired of this; others enjoy it. There are more than 5,000 topics covered, with new ones being added and outdated ones deleted daily. How long the messages stay in the system depends on the system operator; most operators purge old messages every few weeks.

A news reader program is used to access the messages for reading. There are many news readers, each with a different look, that are provided by Internet access providers or that come bundled in Internet software packages. Like mailing lists, Usenet news groups are usually free to the person connected to the Internet.

Usenet groups have a specific hierarchical naming system. The names look odd at first, but the system makes sense once you get the hang of it. The first part of the name describes the general kind of news group, the next part describes the type of group more specifically, and so on. So, for example, groups that start with sci have to do with science; sci.med groups are those related to the medical sciences. The nursing discussion is located at sci.med.nursing to many nurses' dismay. However, the naming has nothing to do with the role of nursing as related to the role of medicine, and it is not an attempt to disempower nurses. It only relates to science, then medical sciences, then nursing. A listing of the top level names of several Usenet groups are presented in Display 3-2.

If you are searching for nursing- and health-related discussions, your best bet is to look in the sci.med groups and the alt.support groups. The sci.med groups are generally discussions among health professionals; the alt.support groups include a wide range of participants, including patients, their families, and health-care providers. Before you use information from a group discussion, or before you refer a patient or colleague to a discussion, be sure to check it out and satisfy your-

---

DISPLAY 3-2. TOP-LEVEL NAMES OF USENET GROUPS

alt
Alternative groups. Setting up a group in any of the following hierarchies is an involved process, requiring a charter and online vote. Anyone can set up an alt group. Many times after it has been around for a while, the readers will pursue having it become a mainstream group, although there are many alt groups that have been around for years and show no evidence of changing.

comp
Topics dealing with computers.

sci
Topics dealing with the sciences.

sci.med
Medical- and health-related science discussions.

rec
Recreational newsgroups, including sports, hobbies, and the arts.

soc
Social newsgroups, including social interests and socializing.

news
Topics having to do with Internet news itself.

talk
Long arguments, frequently political.

self in your own mind that the information is indeed what you expect and need. This is important because many of your patients may find their way to some of the patient support groups. Perhaps you are a diabetes educator. Although you may choose not to refer patients or clients to alt.support.diabetes, if you have computer-literate patients, they may find the group on their own. You would be wise to visit the group, follow the discussions, and assess the information so that if you are asked about it, you can given an informed answer about the content that is available.

The World Wide Web

HISTORY AND OVERVIEW

E-mail lets you communicate with others, either individually or in groups via mailing lists. As noted earlier, this a major portion of the traffic on the Internet. Usenet groups are also forums for discussion. The last major component is the World Wide Web, or WWW, or Web for short. The Web is less interactive than e-mail and exists more as an information provider. You can visit Websites, download files, or search for information, all from the comfort of your personal computer. Recent changes and innovations to the Web have made searching and navigation easier than ever before, which has resulted in a worldwide Internet boom.

In fact, the WWW has grown exponentially since it was first created in 1993. The Web, as we know it today, was created at the European Centre of Particle Physics (CERN) in Switzerland. These are the same folks who developed the universal resource locator (URL). As you browse through some of the more peculiar sites on the Web, you may begin to wonder about the connection between the WWW and its physicist-creators in Switzerland.

As scientists engaged in research, they were constantly accessing and sharing files and data on the Internet and had been for years. But by 1989, the Internet had become unwieldy, even for them, the experienced users. The physicists were finding they were wasting valuable time navigating the Internet; this was cutting into the time available to them for their research. They decided to create an environment in which information of any type from any source could be accessed in a simple and consistent way. Their vision became the Web.

The key features distinguishing the Web from the rest of the Internet are hypertext and multimedia capabilities. E-mail, which was discussed in the previous section, is text based. On the other hand, the Web is full of color, pictures, sound, movies, and music. These are the features that have caught the public's attention and have in large part contributed to the phenomenal growth of the Web.

When you visit a Website, the first thing you'll see is the *home page* for that site. A home page is analogous to a welcome mat. Figure 3-5 is a picture of the Nursing Center home page. A home page typically includes information about the site, why it was created, what is available, and who to contact with comments or ques-

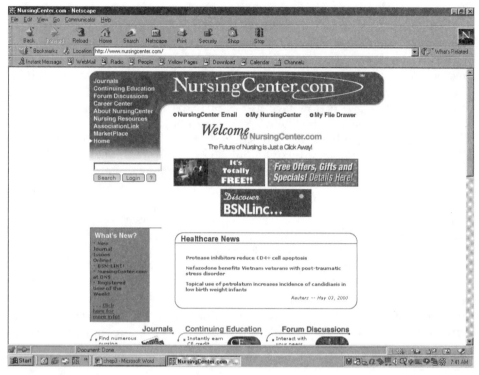

FIGURE 3-5. NursingCenter.com home page.

tions. Home pages often include a running tally of the number of visitors (hits) and the date when the page was last updated.

The language used to create a Web page, *hypertext markup language* (HTML), has several advantages to developers and users. First, HTML can hold text formatting, which allows the designer to incorporate creative design elements into the page. This makes the page easy to read and attractive to look at. Second, HTML provides the ability to create hypertext links to other documents. As you move your cursor over highlighted areas within a WWW document, you'll see it turn into a hand or an arrow. By clicking on this area, using either a mouse or keystroke, another document will be retrieved and opened. This second document may be located in a completely different place on the Internet. Although the document could be on a computer in a remote part of the world, its physical location is irrelevant to you, the user. From the new document, you can click again to continue your exploration. Each of these clicks are called *links*. As you travel the Internet using WWW links, you may end up in a different place, both conceptually and physically, from where you started.

With the proper helper applications, multimedia capabilities add a new dimension to Internet exploration. Graphics, sounds, and movie clips can be incorporated into a Website. Although some of these sites are just plain fun (such as TV theme songs),[1] there are also useful applications of multimedia. I recently met a faculty member who found a Quicktime animation of plaque building up on the arteries of the heart. She incorporated the video into a multimedia class presentation on coronary artery disease. Although the animation was only about 10 seconds long, it clearly demonstrated for students a concept that is often difficult to visualize. One of my favorite sound clips is a recording of Florence Nightingale, yes, the real FN. She made a 52-second recording on July 30, 1890. This recording was made on a cylinder that was discovered and restored in 1939. The recording is available at the Nightingale Museum in London, but it is also available to you on the Internet at the InterNurse site (www.internurse.com).

ACCESS

To access the Web, you need a browser. The original browser, Mosaic, was developed at the National Center for Supercomputing Applications (NCSA) in Illinois. It was available as freeware over the Internet and came in Windows and Macintosh versions. One of the developers of Mosaic left NCSA, started Netscape Communications Corporation, and developed Netscape Navigator. The newest version of this program is now called Communicator. This program, like Mosaic, comes in both Windows and Macintosh versions. Microsoft has also developed a browser, Internet Explorer. Netscape and Internet Explorer are fighting it out for user popularity and have been for quite a few years; it remains to be seen which one will emerge as number one. The recent legal battles for Microsoft will also likely have an impact on the future face of browsers.

Commercial services also provide access to the Web. If you have an account on America Online, for example, you can access the Web using its proprietary Web browser. AT&T WorldNet service uses a modified version of Communicator; RoadRunner from Time Warner Cable uses a modified version of Internet Explorer. It is possible to have more than one browser on your computer, provided you have sufficient room on the hard drive. You are also not required to use a browser that comes with an ISP. For example, if you are an America Online customer, you can connect to America Online, minimize the browser they provide, and start your preferred browser, such as Communicator. Experiment with different programs to find out which one best meets your needs.

As noted in Chapter 2, to use any of these browsers satisfactorily, you must have an Internet connection through a local area network (LAN), modem, cable modem, or other connection, and a relatively high-end computer.

GETTING AROUND

To be able to explore the Internet effectively, the first step is to learn how to use your browser efficiently. An important note to keep in mind is that even though

---

[1]There are TV theme song pages scattered all over the Internet, but one that is fairly comprehensive and seems to be updated regularly can be found at http:/www.classic-tv.com.

there are a number of different browsers available, they all work in a similar fashion. If you learn how to use one browser well, you will be able to easily transfer those skills to another browser. Figure 3-6 is an illustration of the two most popular browsers, Communicator and Internet Explorer. Let's look at the "Navigation Toolbar," which is the horizontal bar at the top with the icons "back," "search," "stop," and so on. Notice that between the two browsers, the functions are similar but the icons and words used to illustrate the functions are slightly different, such as "refresh" in Explorer and "reload" in Communicator. Both of these buttons achieve the same result; that is, causing the page you are viewing to reload.

Getting around requires some basic navigation skills. The "back" and "forward" buttons are very handy; using these buttons will step you back (or forward), page by page, to the sites you have visited. It is very easy, when you are using links on different pages, to go click, click, click, and suddenly be lost! Clicking the back button in essence helps you undo the traveling that you have done.

Another handy feature is to click on the arrow at the end of the URL location bar (see Fig. 3-7). This opens a history of the places you have recently visited. You can quickly move to a prior location by choosing the URL off the drop-down menu that is presented. This same task can be accomplished by clicking on the

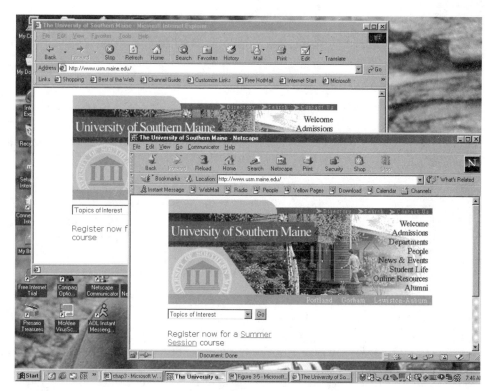

FIGURE 3-6. Illustration of Netscape Communicator and Internet Explorer.

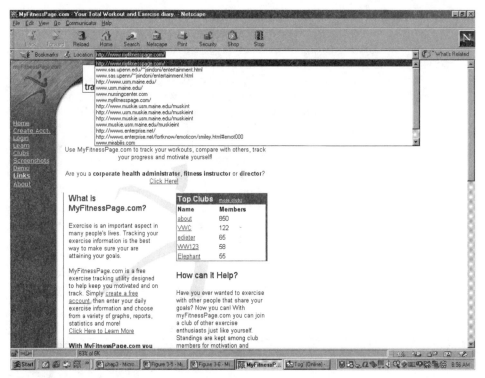

FIGURE 3-7. History of places visited on the URL bar.

"Go" button (see Fig. 3-8). Once again, a history list is presented from which you can select a specific location.

I call the "Home" button the "Wizard of Oz" button. If you get totally lost on the Internet, clicking this button is the same as Dorothy clicking her heels three times—you will immediately go home. You can make this button more useful by making "Home" a place that is meaningful to you. By default, the home button will be preprogrammed, either by your ISP or the browser manufacturer. Thus, in a generic version of Communicator, the default home location is Netscape Communications. Although I have nothing against Netscape, I have reset my home page to be "My Fitness Page" (www.myfitnesspage.com), a site that allows me to log in my daily walk and exercise. Having my walking log come up first thing every morning is a great motivator to keep on track to meet my exercise goals!

To change your home page in Communicator, click on "edit," then "preferences." You will see the page illustrated in Figure 3-9. Simply type in the URL for your desired home page and close the screen by clicking OK. In Explorer, the process is similar: Select "tools," then "Internet options," and type in the URL. You can make any site your home page: your local newspaper, to get the headlines every morning; your workplace or school; or a favorite shopping site. It is also

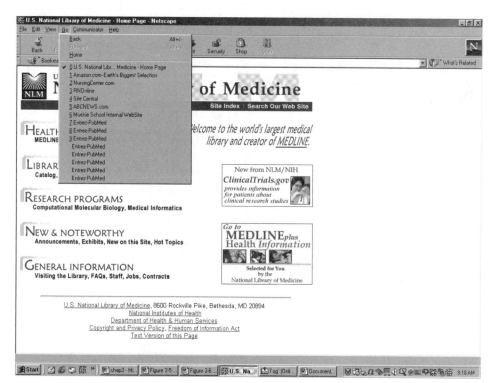

FIGURE 3-8. History of places visited on the Go menu.

possible to leave the home page blank (this is an option on both Communicator and Explorer). If you have a slow modem connection, leaving the home page blank will speed up the initial loading of your browser.

Finally, remember that there are usually several ways to do the same thing. That is, you can navigate using the buttons on the navigation toolbar; you can use commands on the drop-down menus; and you can use a combination of key-strokes, such as "Alt-Home," to go home. Investigate your browser, open the drop-down menus, and play around with different features to learn how to make your Internet travel quick and efficient.

Tips for Using Search Engines to Explore the Internet

Search engines are tools that enable you to expand from finding a single source of information (one Website) to locating several sites related to a single subject. There are many different search engines available on the Internet. Unfortunately, none of them are perfect. A study published in *Science* in 1998[1] revealed that even the best search engines found approximately 33% of the information available on the Web. That, of course, means that 67% of useful information is being missed.

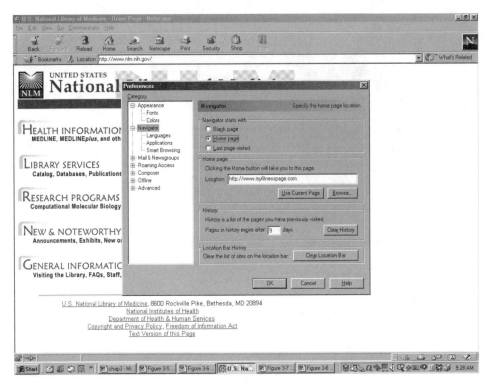

FIGURE 3-9. Changing your home page location (Communicator).

Search engines are good starting points, and you can maximize their effectiveness by considering the following suggestions. But keep in mind that you will also want to use other methods to find the information you need on the Web.

First, identify your search. Are you looking for broad information on cancer, or are you looking for patient education resources to recommend to breast cancer patients? Narrowing the topic of your search as much as possible will help you to search the Internet more efficiently. Know exactly what it is you are searching for before you start your search.

Choose the right search engine. There are many popular search engines, such as AltaVista, InfoSeek, WebCrawler, Yahoo, and HotBot. All have features that distinguish themselves from each other. If you use AltaVista, you can scour the Internet for the most obscure resources, but you may have to pull information out from among 10,000 other found references (called *hits*). Yahoo allows you to search using defined categories that will usually render fewer hits, but you may miss some important information. Try the same search in a variety of search engines and see what you retrieve. This is a good way to become familiar with the different engines and what they are able to offer you.

There are also mega-search engines; that is, search engines that search a variety of search engines. Metacrawler (www.metacrawler.com) and Dogpile (www.dogpile.com) are two reliable ones. Again, try the same search in each and compare the results to get a flavor of what they can offer you.

Select the keywords for your search carefully. Obviously, if you are looking for breast cancer information, the words "breast" and "cancer" should be among the keywords you choose. However, if those are the only words you use and you are searching with AltaVista, you'll have 70,000 hits to pore through. To make this search more efficient, ask yourself "Breast cancer information in relation to what?" Choosing additional keywords such as "organizations," "Usenet," and "support" will help you to narrow your search to a manageable number of hits.

Learn to use the features of the search engine to narrow your search. If you need the most up-to-date information, you may define a specific time period in the search field. You may be able to use advanced query language (also called *Boolean searches*) such as "and," "not," and "or" to define your search. You might want to search only Websites or Usenet groups. Take advantage of these features and save yourself valuable time.

Brute Force Works, Too

Search engines work very well, especially when you know exactly what you are looking for. For example, I recently wanted to find out how many people died in airplane crashes in 1999. With a focused search and careful selection of key words, I had the answer in 5 minutes. However, sometimes a search engine is not giving you what you need. This generally happens when I want more general information. In this case, I often revert to the "brute force" method of Internet exploration.

With brute force, try typing in an address and see what you get. The worst that can happen is that you will get an annoying message telling you the site cannot be found. Think of how the addresses work: most start with www and end with a domain name. Perhaps you are trying to find a School of Nursing, let's say at the University of New Hampshire, popularly known as UNH. Typing **http://www.unh.edu** will take you right to the university, and from there, you can find the link to the Nursing Department home page. If your first guess doesn't work, try another: **http://www.acs.org** will take you to the American Chemical Society, but **http://www.cancer.org** takes you to the American Cancer Society.

Take Advantage of Links and Use the Bookmark Feature

Every single Website has links to other Websites of related interest. Take advantage of these links because the site developer has already done some of the work of finding other useful resources. Once again, combine brute force and links to get the information you need. Using breast cancer as an example, you might start at the American Cancer Society. There is a lot of information right at the site, but you can also connect to the following:

- Oncolink, at the University of Pennsylvania
- National Breast Cancer Coalition
- Nysernet Breast Cancer Information Clearinghouse
- National Cancer Institute

These are just a few of the links available from the ACS. Each site you visit will have more links, and in this way, the resources keep building. I generally find that this approach works well when I am less focused in the information I need. Visiting a variety of sites will open up the vistas of information available. When you find a site that has useful information, be sure to bookmark it. On more than one occasion, I have been unable to easily return to a site of interest because I can't remember how I got there in the first place and I neglected to add a bookmark to my list.

PUTTING THE PIECES TOGETHER TO BECOME AN INSTANT EXPERT

This discussion has given you the basic tools you need to move around on the Web and search for and find useful information. I often say that the Internet has opened up a world of information so that anyone can become an instant expert on a given topic in 15 minutes or less. Although that might be a slight exaggeration, it is not entirely false. Every time I go online to find information on a new subject, I use the following approach:

1. First, what is your topic of interest? At this point, you can be very broad; I have done searches on topics as general as "menopause" or "composting toilets."
2. Do a "quick and dirty" search on the topic. I personally like AltaVista (www.altavista.com), but any search engine will do.
3. You'll probably get an enormous number of hits, but start with the first 10 or so on the list. Look at the URLs and try to decipher where they are. Pay attention to the domains; "com" is going to be a commercial site, so that may be a business related to your topic. "Edu" is an educational institution.
4. Quickly visit a few sites. Look for the information you need, or useful links. If a site is not relevant, use the back button to return to your search results and go to the next site.

By clicking and linking, I have found that I can get a starting handle on the information I need in a relatively short period of time. An alternate to this approach is to use the "brute force" method in step one; that is, if you know of a site that is relevant to your topic, start your search there. For example, the Agency for Healthcare Research and Quality has good links on clinical practice guidelines, so if I am looking for information on evidence-based practice, I will often start my search by simply typing in **www.ahrq.gov**.

Gopher

The WWW as we know it today was developed between 1989 and 1993 at CERN and has become the dominant force on the Internet. Before the graphical user interface of the WWW, much of the Internet was text-based and difficult to navigate. To address that situation, the Microcomputer, Workstation and Networks Center at the University of Minnesota made the first serious attempt to bring a simple, practical user interface to the Internet with their development of Gopher software, which was introduced in 1991. The name was a bit of a joke: the software "goes for" (go-fer) your files. The University of Minnesota is also the home of the Golden Gophers. The software was made available free to educational institutions throughout the world. Because of their ease of use, Gopher servers rapidly spread throughout the Internet after the software was introduced.

In earlier editions of this book, I included many Gopher sites, because they were quite common. With this edition, they have all more or less disappeared. But I include this brief comment in case you happen to stumble upon an older Gopher server. If you access a Gopher site through a browser, it is easily recognizable from the series of folders that will be presented on your screen. Internet Gophers are information servers that present you with a hierarchical menu of resources in a simple, consistent manner. At a Gopher site, Internet navigation becomes a matter of reading menus, as opposed to clicking on graphical icons.

As an interesting historical tidbit, one of the first nursing Gophers was the Nightingale Gopher at the University of Tennessee. This site was very well done with a wealth of information about conferences, people, and clinical issues. The site has been changed over to a Website and the Gopher files are no longer available. Even so, we should remember the pioneering role that the Nightingale Gopher took when it first sought to organize and present nursing information to a wide audience of users.

Being Realistic: What to Expect on Your Internet Journey

So far, I have covered how to travel and what to see on the Internet. Are you ready to venture forth? Probably, but I want to include a few words of warning about what you can and cannot expect on your journey. I have friends who have traveled to Jamaica, expecting a tropical paradise, but have been shocked to discover the poverty that exists in that small island nation. The Internet is the same way. As you prepare for your journey, keep the following in mind.

WHAT TO EXPECT

The first thing to expect on your Internet journey is confusion. People have described the Internet as the modern equivalent of the Wild West frontier and at times that seems to be an apt description. Although things are becoming more organized out there in the Internet world, a high degree of confusion still exists.

Give yourself some time to learn your way around and discover how to best find the information you are seeking. Do not expect to become an expert overnight. I have been at this for several years now, and some days, I still feel like a novice.

Prepare yourself for lots of irrelevant material. In discussion groups, for example, people have a way of getting off track. Although the header says "Breast cancer research results," the message might not have anything to do with breast cancer or research. It is common to hear people discuss the "high signal-to-noise ratio" on the Internet. This simply means that for every useful bit of information you find, you'll have to sift through an equal number of useless bits.

You can also expect to find a virtual community. This is one of the pleasant surprises of the Internet. Although there are millions of people accessing the Internet every day, you'll quickly learn the names and personalities of the members of your Internet world. In particular, I have found that nurses on the Internet are a very friendly group. As a group, we tend to be quick to offer help, answer questions, share experiences, and talk about nursing. Nurses on the Internet are tolerant of newbies (those new to the Net), keep flaming to a minimum (especially compared to some of the more virulent groups), and are even accepting of NRNs.[2] Clinicians, researchers, teachers, administrators, and many nurses from around the globe form our virtual community.

The Internet is a great leveler. You are interacting with people in nontraditional ways. Issues that sometimes get in the way of traditional communication, such as gender, skin color, height, or weight, become irrelevant on the Internet. People are free to have open, honest discussions. Of course, having these discussions is a special privilege. Respect the time and information that people share with you and do not trivialize their contributions.

Finally, things happen quickly on the Internet. You can post a question and may have several answers within minutes. Be prepared for this both in terms of receiving and responding to messages. I occasionally post requests to the nurse educators discussion group asking for software reviewers for *Computers in Nursing*. Replies have come back to me in as little as 60 seconds! I learned very quickly not to post such a request on a day when I would not be in my office and able to check my e-mail at frequent intervals.

WHAT NOT TO EXPECT

Just as you can expect to find a wealth of useful information, there are certain things you should not expect on the Internet. Many people begin their journey with unrealistic expectations and then are disappointed when the trip does not deliver. Here are a few things to remember as you begin your journey.

You Will Not Find Full Text. In fact, that is not entirely true. You will find some full text, but not all of the items you might want in full text will be available. Nurses want full text of journal articles, nursing texts, patient education materials, and

---

[2]NRN stands for "not an RN"; that is, a person who is not a nurse. Gary Hales, founding editor of *Computers in Nursing*, is credited with coining this term.

the like. For the most part, these types of materials are available in a limited way on the Internet.

There are online searching services, such as Internet Grateful Med (IGM; http://igm.nlm.nih.gov), that will allow you to search for journal citations in the MEDLINE database of the National Library of Medicine (NLM). Approximately 70% of the entries in MEDLINE include abstracts, and they can be retrieved using IGM. You can use Loansome Doc to order the articles from a cooperating library, but you cannot find the full text of articles online through MEDLINE. The National Library of Medicine has developed a new service, PUBMED, that has full text available for a limited number of articles, but there are fees associated with accessing this information. Another example is the UnCover database from CARL. Searching is free, but if you want an article, you pay for the document delivery service. A colleague recently described these systems as menus in a restaurant: they don't charge you to read the menu, but they charge you when they bring you your food.

At the NursingCenter (www.nursingcenter.com), it is possible to find full text of recent articles from some of their journals, such as the *American Journal of Nursing* and *Computers in Nursing*. Abstracts of the articles are available online; if you want the full text, there is a fee. If you do a literature search and need an older article, you will need to rely on traditional retrieval methods, such as a trip to the library or interlibrary loan.

At the site for the Agency for Healthcare Research and Quality (AHRQ; http://www.ahrq.gov/), you can search and download full text of their clinical practice guidelines. This is an example of full text that is available and is certainly a useful resource to know about. Of course, a major advantage of the online version is the ability to search the document. The online version also includes hypertext links to the references in the guideline. Both of these features are useful and unavailable in the printed version. Several medical journals, such as *JAMA*, also have full text available at the Websites (jama.ama-assn.org). Unfortunately, the availability of resources such as these is sporadic; there is no consistency at this time about what is available and what is not. In terms of finding literature resources, don't abandon the library just yet. You will probably still need to use the trusty copier and printed journals on occasion.

Not Everything Is Free. Remember the expression, "There is no such thing as a free lunch"? This is often true on the Internet. Although the Internet was designed from its roots to be a noncommercial service, that does not mean all Internet resources are free. You may need to pay or subscribe to obtain access to certain services. For example, *Online Journal of Knowledge Synthesis for Nursing* (www.stti.iupui.edu/library/ojksn/) requires a subscription (currently $90 to $105 per year) for access. If you are not a subscriber, you will not be able to access the journal. Although subscribing to journals in the non-Internet world is commonplace, many people are surprised when they encounter it on the Internet.

Many sites require registration to access their features, but there is no charge for the registration. This allows the site developers to learn more about who is visiting the site and what information they desire. Once you have registered, many sites will give you the option of receiving regular e-mail updates about site changes and other news of interest.

Evaluating What You Find

The final element in being an effective Internet traveler is having the ability to evaluate the information that you find. Just as you would use your critical thinking skills as a nurse to evaluate a print document, so must you evaluate the information you find on the Web. The Internet is a wonderful resource but that does not mean that all the resources on the Web are wonderful!

Over my years of Internet searching, I have developed some personal criteria for evaluation, which I have found have served me well. Recently, a student[3] suggested a useful mnemonic, "Are you PLEASED with the site?" which I have adapted to fit my existing criteria. To determine if you are PLEASED, consider the following:

- **P**—Purpose
  What is the author's purpose in developing the site? Are the author's objectives clear? Many people will develop a Website as a hobby or a way of sharing information they have gathered. I look at this type of a site very differently than a site that has been developed as a commercial service, selling a product or resource. It should be immediately evident to you what is the true purpose of the site.
- **L**—Links
  Evaluate the links at the site. Are they working? Links that don't take you anywhere are called "dead links." Do they link to reliable sites? It is important to critically evaluate the links at sites hosted by organizations, businesses, or institutions because these entities are usually presenting themselves as authorities for the subject at hand. Many times, they will include a blanket disclaimer such as "Organization X assumes no responsibility for the credibility or authority of the following links." I consider that hogwash. If an organization is devoting time and resources to creating a Web page, then part of that responsibility is to ensure that the links they provide go to sources they deem credible and reliable. I have little patience with organizations that include "laundry lists" of links, many of which prove to be dubious or unreliable.

    Some pages, such as those created by individuals, are really nothing more than a collection of links. These can be useful as a starting point for a search, but it is still important to evaluate the links that are provided at the site.
- **E**—Editorial (site content)
  Is the information contained in the site accurate, comprehensive, and current? Is there a particular bias, or is the information presented in an objec-

[3]Thanks to Linda Johnson, of Regents College in Albany, NY, for her original suggestion of this mnemonic.

tive way? Also assess who is the consumer of the site: is it designed for health professionals, patients, consumers or other audiences?

- **A—Author**
  Who is the author of the site? Does that person or persons have the appropriate credentials? Is the author clearly identified by name, and is contact information provided? Many times, I will double-check on an author's credentials by doing a literature search in MEDLINE (using GratefulMed or PubMed). When a person advertises him or herself as "the leading worldwide authority" on such-and-such topic, I figure he or she should have a few publications to his or her credit that establishes his or her reputation.

- **S—Site**
  Is the site easy to navigate? Is it attractive? Does it download quickly or have too many graphics and other features that make it inefficient? A site that is pleasing to the eye will invite you to return. Sites that cause my computer to crash go on the "never visit again" list. I am also not fond of sites that have annoying music that cannot be turned off.

- **E—Ethical**
  Is there contact information for the site developer and author? Is there full disclosure of who the author is and the purpose of the site? Is this information easy to find, or is it buried deep in the Website? There are many commercial services, particularly pharmaceutical companies, that have excellent Websites with very useful information. But some of them exist only to sell their product, although this is not immediately evident. I consider this an ethical violation.

- **D—Date**
  When was the site last updated? Is it current? Is the information something that needs to be updated regularly? Generally, with health and nursing information, the answer to the last question is yes. I become concerned with sites that have not been updated within 12 to 18 months. The date the site was last updated should be prominently displayed on the site. Keep in mind that different pages within the site may be updated at different times. Be sure to check the date on each of the pages that you visit.

Health On the Net Foundation

There are many resources available on the WWW for evaluation criteria, both for health-related sites as well as general sites. One source that I have found to be consistently reliable is the Health On the Net Foundation (www.hon.ch). The following brief history is presented at its Website:

> Health On the Net Foundation's origins go back to September 7-8, 1995, when some of the world's foremost experts on telemedicine gathered in Geneva, Switzerland, for a conference entitled The Use of the Internet and World Wide Web for Telematics in Healthcare. The 60 participants came from 11 countries. They included U.S. heart surgeon Dr. Michael DeBakey, physicians and professors, researchers and senior representatives of the World Health Organisation (WHO), International Telecommunication

Union (ITU), the European Laboratory for Particle Physics (CERN), the European Commission, the National Library of Medicine and the G7-Global Healthcare Applications Project. As the conference wound up, they unanimously voted to create a permanent body that would, in the words of the programme, "promote the effective and reliable

---

DISPLAY 3-3. HEALTH ON THE NET FOUNDATION CODE OF CONDUCT FOR MEDICAL WEB SITES

Principle 1: Authority
Any medical or health advice provided and hosted on this site will only be given by medically trained and qualified professionals unless a clear statement is made that a piece of advice offered is from a non-medically qualified individual or organisation.

Principle 2: Complementarity
The information provided on this site is designed to support, not replace, the relationship that exists between a patient/site visitor and his/her existing physician.

Principle 3: Confidentiality
Confidentiality of data relating to individual patients and visitors to a medical/health Web site, including their identity, is respected by this Web site. The Web site owners undertake to honour or exceed the legal requirements of medical/health information privacy that apply in the country and state where the Web site and mirror sites are located.

Principle 4: Attribution
Where appropriate, information contained on this site will be supported by clear references to source data and, where possible, have specific HTML links to that data. The date when a clinical page was last modified will be clearly displayed (e.g. at the bottom of the page).

Principle 5: Justifiability
Any claims relating to the benefits/performance of a specific treatment, commercial product or service will be supported by appropriate, balanced evidence in the manner outlined above in Principle 4.

Principle 6: Transparency of Authorship
The designers of this Web site will seek to provide information in the clearest possible manner and provide contact addresses for visitors that seek further information or support. The Webmaster will display his/her E-mail address clearly throughout the Web site.

Principle 7: Transparency of Sponsorship
Support for this Web site will be clearly identified, including the identities of commercial and non-commercial organisations that have contributed funding, services or material for the site.

Principle 8: Honesty in Advertising and Editorial Policy
If advertising is a source of funding it will be clearly stated. A brief description of the advertising policy adopted by the Web site owners will be displayed on the site. Advertising and other promotional material will be presented to viewers in a manner and context that facilitates differentiation between it and the original material created by the institution operating the site.

Source: Health On the Net Foundation, http://www.hon.ch/HONcode/Conduct.html

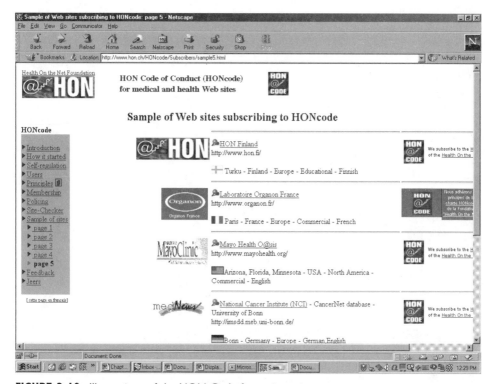

FIGURE 3-10. Illustrations of the HON Code for various sites.

use of the new technologies for telemedicine in healthcare around the world." HON's site went live some six months later. On March 20, 1996, www.hon.ch became one of the very first URLs to guide both lay users and medical professionals to reliable sources of healthcare information in cyberspace.

An early and ongoing intiative of the HON Foundation was to create the HON Code of Conduct for the Web. The principles of this code are presented in Display 3-3. Users and Website developers who abide by the HON Code are invited to display the HON symbol, which is illustrated in Figure 3-10. A site must go through a registration and approval process to display the code and, in doing so, agree to abide by the principles of the HON Foundation. Even when you see the symbol displayed, it is still a good idea to verify the accuracy of the site, so that you can be confident in your own mind that it is what it purports to be.

REFERENCE

1. Lawrence S, Giles CL. Searching the World Wide Web. *Science* 1998; April 3;280:98–100.

CHAPTER 4

■■

Entertaining Diversions for the Internet Traveler

The purpose of this book has been to provide a professional guide to Internet travel, but even folks on business trips can take an afternoon off for sight-seeing or other diversions. The Internet is no exception: shopping, chatting, and making friends online are all popular activities for Internet explorers. This chapter provides a brief overview of some of the more popular leisure pursuits available on the Internet.

SHOPPING ON THE WEB[1]

No doubt about it, shopping on the Internet is wildly popular and the number two reason that many people decide to get online (e-mail is number one). During the 1999 holiday season, online sales swelled to more than double those of holiday season 1998. The US government estimated online retail sales at $5.3 billion, which, as impressive as it sounds, was only 0.6 percent of total sales in the United States for the fourth quarter of 1999. Television news reports estimated that approximately 24 percent of all holiday shoppers had used the Internet to purchase at least one gift. In many ways, the Internet is beginning to resemble a giant mall, to the dismay of many of the original developers of the Web.

---

[1]The section on "Shopping on the Web" was adapted from "E-commerce: A Quick Guide to Online Shopping," written by Susan Shropshire and published in *CIN Plus*, vol. 3, no. 2, May 1, 2000, pp. 4, 10, 12.

Is online shopping safe? Although most of us don't think twice about handing a credit card to a waitperson or reading it over the phone to a catalog order taker, many are still reluctant to shop on the Web. In any situation, it is possible that the card information could be stolen and used fraudulently. Although entering name, address, and credit card information on a blank form at a Website can seem as though you're revealing personal information that anyone might pick up, the risks of online shopping are basically the same as those encountered in everyday purchases.

Anatomy of an E-transaction

How does the information get safely to the merchant? Who's on the other end— can they be trusted to keep information private, as well as to honor the transaction? How can you tell, if you can't see or speak to a real person?

When you access a merchant's site, and particularly if you select items for purchase (whether or not you actually complete the transaction), your browser will probably accept a cookie from the server hosting the merchant's Website. If you decide to buy, you should be guided to a secure connection on the host server so that the privacy of the transaction is ensured; no one can "eavesdrop" on the conversation. There are a number of ways to check on the merchant itself. If you're armed with the right information, you can safely shop on the Internet.

Cookies

If you've ever seen something like, "Greetings, Mary Jones!" on your second visit to a Website, it means the server hosting the Web page has placed what is known as a cookie on the hard drive of your computer. Internet cookies are small data files used by Web servers to identify Web users. Popular rumors credit cookies with the ability to gather all sorts of information about you—passwords, credit card numbers, a listing of all the software resident on your hard drive— but the true nature of an Internet cookie is far less sinister.

There are two types of cookies. The more common kind is destroyed when you quit your browser; the second type, known as a persistent cookie, comes with an expiration date, and is stored on your hard drive until the date passes. Both kinds can be used to track browsing habits (for example, if you visit an online pet store and identify yourself as a ferret owner, the next time you visit, thanks to the cookie, you may be presented with a coupon for ferret supplies). However, because cookies are data files and not segments of code that can direct the operation of your computer, they are basically only "convenience handles" used to identify patrons. All of the information transmitted via cookies is gathered and stored in Web server data logs, whether or not cookies are accepted by your browser. Most of the time, cookies simply make it easier for Web providers to extract certain types of information (such as Internet Protocol [IP] address, browser type, and computer operating system).

SHOPPING CARTS AND HOME PAGES

If your browser has accepted a cookie from a site, a copy is returned to the server whenever a file is requested. This is how shopping carts work; the server collects information about whatever merchandise is added to the shopping cart identified by your cookie, and can tally subtotals, tax, and shipping costs for that particular order.

Similarly, cookies are used to build customized home pages. Your browser will accept a cookie for each of the items you request to have displayed on your home page; every time you log in, the browser will send that set of cookies to the Web server, and the server will display the selected items.

ARE COOKIES BAD FOR YOU?

Cookies do have a less benign use: on multiple-client sites serviced by a single marketer, one cookie can be used to build a profile on a single user. If the client sites reference the marketer's advertisement with a tag that points to a URL, the advertiser can easily send your browser a cookie when you open the client site's page, and that cookie will be returned to the advertiser any time you open a page that displays one of their ads. While this probably results in a scattershot picture rather than an invasive, Big Brother-style profile of your Internet use— the marketer can't tell what you do when you open the page, only how many times you access it and what the IP address of your computer is—it can be used to build an e-mail address list targeting you for unsolicited commercial e-mail, or spam.

CRUMBLING COOKIES

You can examine and even remove persistent cookies by opening the files placed in your browser's cookie directory. Netscape Communicator stores persistent cookies in a personal computer (PC) file called cookies.txt; Microsoft's Internet Explorer stores them in a cookies directory located under Windows. If you delete a cookie that you had wanted to keep, the worst that can happen is the next time you visit your favorite site, you'll be treated as a new user.

You can also prevent your browser from accepting cookies by accessing the options menu and directing it to disable cookies, or you can have it prompt you whenever a site attempts to send a cookie to you. Think twice before you implement either of these choices, since you'll probably spend a fair amount of time answering dialog boxes, either to identify yourself as a user or to accept or deny cookies, while you surf.

There are also cookie-blocking software programs available that can instruct your Web browser to accept cookies only from designated sites, which is really convenient if you have a favorite, trusted Internet merchant. Check out the Junkbusters site (www.junkbusters.com) or Cookie Central (www.cookiecentral.com) for more information on these programs.

Security

Recent versions of Netscape Communicator and Internet Explorer, both of which are known as "secure browsers," are capable of transmitting data in protected form so that it can be safely stored on the destination server.

The technology employed in secure communications is called Secure Sockets Layer (SSL) and is a set of rules that include encryption, which prevents unauthorized users from intercepting information; data integrity, which ensures that communications aren't tampered with during transmission; and authentication, which verifies that the party actually receiving your communication is who it claims to be.

How Does Encryption Work?

When data are sent securely, they are scrambled according to a certain "key" that prescribes substitutions, and only a recipient with the right "key" can unscramble the data once received. At present, two levels of encryption are used, 40 bit and 128 bit. 40-bit encryption can use billions of possible keys to decipher the coded information, but with 128-bit encryption, there are 300 billion trillion times as many keys. That's why online banking and financial services usually require you to employ 128-bit encryption: it is virtually impossible for an unauthorized party to find the right key. Even if the information were intercepted, it would arrive as gibberish.

To check a site's security status, look at the site's URL in your browser window. An "s" added to the familiar "http" ("https") shows that SSL is in effect. In earlier versions of Netscape Navigator, a secure site is indicated when the broken key symbol in the lowerleft corner of your browser window becomes solid; in Netscape Communicator 4.0 and later, and in Internet Explorer 4.0, an open padlock symbol closes in secure mode.

Usually, your browser will notify you when you are about to connect to a secure server, and again when you request insecure information (for example, if you view items in your shopping cart, and then decide to return to shopping). SSL protects communications during transmission, but you must also protect yourself by dealing only with legitimate Internet companies.

Authentication

Authentication is provided by services such as VeriSign, who provide verification of site legitimacy. Site certification is a process by which, for a fee, a merchant proves to a central repository that it is who it claims to be and is extended an electronic certificate stating both that fact and the name of the certifier. You can check a site's server certificate by clicking the "Security" button on your browser, then under "Encryption" click "View Certificate." (If "View Certificate" isn't displayed, the site does not have a certificate.)

If you deal with a site whose certificate is not recognized by your browser, you will be prompted by a "wizard" that displays information not only about the company but also about the certifier, and you'll be asked to accept or deny the merchant's ability to transact with you.

Tips to Protect Yourself While Shopping Online

Although shopping online is generally safe and becoming safer every day, even in the online world the caveat is "Buyer beware." Here are a few extra tips to keep in mind as you shop.

Always use the latest version of your browser. Up-to-date browsers contain the latest security technology. Similarly, make sure the site you're purchasing from uses SSL. Check for the "s" after "http," or be sure the key or padlock symbols are closed. Look for symbols of authenticity, such as the VeriSign certificate symbol. Larger, well-known companies are probably more likely to properly secure their sites to protect customers, but any reputable Web merchant should prominently display security information and a privacy policy explaining what information is gathered, how it is used, and how it is protected.

Look for a phone number or e-mail address to contact in case you have questions about anything, including security procedures. You can check out a prospective merchant at sites like e-BuyersGuide.com, which publishes results of consumer surveys and rates confidence in different e-tailers, and also features an interactive US map with links to legal resources in the event you need to report a fraud.

Keep a record. Most e-commerce sites present you with an invoice or transaction summary before you submit your order; many will also confirm the deal with a follow-up e-mail, if you provide an address, and with a shipper's tracking number so that you can anticipate delivery. Print out this invoice or save it as a file to refer to later, if necessary.

One final consideration in making purchases online is form of payment. Most banks and consumer organizations recommend using a credit card, because if the worst happens and someone manages to get your card number and information, credit card companies usually cap the amount you are liable for if you notify them within a certain time period after the information is stolen. Debit cards, money orders, and checks are not covered by the same protections. I know some people who have one credit card they use exclusively for Internet shopping. If anything untoward happens, then that card can immediately be cancelled. Finally, always carefully examine your monthly statements and follow up on purchases that look unfamiliar.

Auctions

There are stores on the Internet, such as amazon.com, and there are auctions. Just like real auctions, you bid on an item, and if you are the highest bidder, you own it! Auctions allow you to find that special collectible, piece of memorabilia, first edition of a book, or just about anything else your heart desires. Auctions can be great fun, and you may be lucky and score a great deal. But once again, be cautious. Keep the following auction shopping tips in mind.

First, make sure you understand exactly how the auction works. There are different types of auctions, and there are differences in how the various services work. Many of the larger auctions have a tutorial or help file that you should read and familiarize yourself with before submitting any bids.

Second, realize that the auction service probably makes little or no attempt to verify the sincerity of the seller's claims. Check out the seller as much as possible. If it is a company, try the Better Business Bureau; if it is an individual, check into his or her feedback section on the auction site. Feedback sections that encourage previous customers to rate sellers (and buyers) are now incorporated into most online auction services. Although feedback sections can be very helpful in establishing a good track record for a seller, you must still be careful. Positive reviews can be faked in some cases, and an empty feedback section is certainly no guarantee that there won't be problems.

Third, be especially skeptical of claims about collectibles, and insist on written appraisals and verifications when appropriate. One of the most common ways that people get ripped off in online auctions is by believing fraudulent claims about authenticity, history, or value of unseen items from unknown sellers.

Fourth, pay by credit card if possible, check if necessary, and never by cash. If you have any problems, make sure and let the auction service know, as well as take the time to describe your experience in the seller's feedback section. A good idea for adding some peace of mind to doing business with strangers, especially when dealing with big ticket items, is to use an online escrow service. Companies like I-Escrow provide this service, in which the buyer sends his payment to the escrow company, then the escrow company tells the seller the payment is in hand and they may deliver the purchased item. The buyer then has a short period of time to approve the purchase and authorize the escrow company to release the money to the seller, or to reject the item and return it to the seller. The escrow service waits until the buyer gives the go-ahead to turn the money over to the seller, or until the seller says he or she has received the returned item, in which case the payment gets returned to the buyer.

DOWNLOADING FILES

Downloading files from the Internet can provide you with games, pictures, clip art, updated drivers for your computer and its accessories, software, programs, and more. You may be shopping, buy a software program, and be asked if you want to download it or have it shipped on CD or disk via the mail. Or, you may have bought a new printer and want to download the latest version of the driver so that it operates correctly with your computer and allows you to take full advantage of all the printer's features. In other words, downloading files from the WWW is quickly becoming a staple of Internet traveling.

Once you begin exploring what can be downloaded, you will be amazed at the wide variety of files that are available on the Internet. Just about anything you can imagine is out there. Don't get carried away, however! Even enormous hard drives run out of room (eventually) and downloaded files can harbor dangerous viruses.

Terms that you will probably come across are freeware and shareware. "Freeware" are files that are available for free. Utilities, drivers, games, and programs are all available for free on the Internet. "Shareware" is a file for which you are requested to make a payment for its use, but you don't need to make the payment at the time you download the file. Shareware allows you to download a program (or something else), evaluate it, and if it is what you were looking for, you can purchase it after evaluation. Many shareware programs work on the honor system: you are expected to make the payment, but if you don't, there is no way that anyone can follow up and force you to do so. Some shareware programs only work in a limited fashion until you make the payment, at which point you are given a key (or something else to unlock the program) for the full version. There are also files available for purchase, for which you must submit payment information before downloading the file. If you choose to purchase software online, keep the shopping tips from the previous section in mind.

Finding Files to Download

Files are available all over the Internet, and finding them does not take too much searching. There are sites that are repositories of files. Two of my favorites are ZDNet (www.zdnet.com) and Cnet (www.cnet.com). If you are looking for drivers for your computer or printer or other accessories, visit the manufacturer's Website.

Many files are compressed, which makes them smaller in size and thus faster to download. WinZip is by far the most popular compression program that is in use today. Files compressed with WinZip have the extension .zip. A compressed file will not work until you decompress it (unzip it, in computer lingo), using the proper decompression software. WinZip is available as shareware ($29 if you decide to keep it) and can be downloaded from both of the sites noted earlier.

As you visit sites with files for downloading, keep your evaluation criteria in mind. Does the site appear to be reputable? Is it a professional and well-maintained site, and is the information up to date? Viruses can be transmitted through downloaded files, and you increase your risk if you download files from amateur, poorly maintained, and disreputable sites.

VIRUSES

Just a brief word on viruses: they are a serious risk and are becoming more so every day. The Internet world was crippled in May 2000 with the "ILOVEYOU" virus that spread all over the world in less than 24 hours. I was the recipient of 37 "ILOVEYOU" messages, but fortunately, I had my wits about me and didn't open any of the attachments; thus, my computer was safe from its attack. I know others who were not as careful and did damage to their own and their companies' systems.

To protect yourself from viruses, practice the basics of safe computing. First, buy a virus-checking program, install it on your computer, and keep it updated. All of the current virus-checking programs have updates available online and most will prompt you when it is time to download an update. Second, if you download files, obtain them from reputable sites. Scan files with your virus checker before opening them. Set your preferences to automatically save files, so that you must open them manually. In your e-mail program, set the preferences so that attachments are not opened automatically but must be opened manually. Third, be suspicious. If you receive an attachment from someone you do not know, investigate it before you open it. If you cannot figure out what the file is or why you would have received it, delete it without opening it. If it is important, the person will send it again. Trust me on this! I have received manuscripts for *Computers in Nursing* that have been sent as attachments without a "cover e-mail" or other identifying information. Files like that go right into my trash bin. Weeks later, I might get a phone call from the author inquiring about the status of the manuscript, and I promptly inform him or her that anonymous attachments are not accepted by *Computers in Nursing*. Although my attitude may seem harsh to some, I have too much valuable information on my computer to risk its being destroyed by a malicious virus. Finally, be observant. Multiple e-mail messages from people you do not know, with the same subject line, should alert you that something fishy is going on.

The Mechanics of Downloading a File

Before you begin downloading, I recommend that you create a new folder (directory) on your hard drive for temporary download files. The biggest problem that most people seem to have is that the file gets downloaded and then "lost" on their hard drive. They do not know what the file is named or where it is located. If you have a download directory (name it something clever, like DOWNLOAD) where you save all downloaded files, then you will always know where they are.

Once you have done that, follow these six steps to successfully download the file from the Web:

1. Go to the Web page that contains the link to the file you wish to download.
2. Click on the download link (usually a link that says "Download" or the name of the file).
3. Indicate which language and operating system you use, if necessary.
4. Select the download site nearest to you, if given a choice. A window will pop up asking whether you wish to open the file or save it to disk.
5. Select "Save to disk" to retain the file for future use. If you want to use it only once, select "Open."
6. If you selected "Save to disk," choose where you want the file to be located on your hard disk; that is, your newly created DOWNLOAD directory.

Most browsers then open a window indicating download progress, including percentage downloaded and time remaining. Note: You can still browse the Web while your file is downloading. Just click on the original browser window. You can begin using the file as soon as the download has finished, if it is not a compressed file. If it is, you must decompress it before you can use it.

Many browsers offer the option of downloading multiple files simultaneously. However, downloading multiple files at once takes just as long as downloading them one at a time. Also, be aware that large files can take a long time to download, especially if you have a slow connection via a modem.

CHATTING ONLINE

As discussed in Chapter 3, mailing lists are one way to meet people with similar interests and have ongoing discussions. But mailing lists are asynchronous—you are not conversing in real time with someone else. If you want to have a synchronous conversation with another person, you need to find a way to chat.

Internet chatting is becoming as popular as e-mail. There are literally hundreds of chat rooms scattered all over the Internet, with people talking on every imaginable topic. Like mailing lists, chat rooms appeal to some, and not at all to others. The only way to find out if online chatting is your idea of fun is to dive in and try it.

To get started, you have two major options: one is to find a chat room that exists on the Internet and go into the chat room and begin conversing; the other option is to download software that allows you to chat, such as Internet relay chat (IRC) or ICQ. Many people (myself included) use both options. People tend to have favorites, so you may find certain online friends in ICQ, others on IRC, and yet others in chat rooms on America Online.

No matter which option you choose, certain rules of etiquette govern chatting. You should also observe certain precautions to protect yourself. One rule to follow: never give out personal information in a chat room. For example; if you're in a chat room and someone claiming to be an official of some sort asks for credit card information or your password, do not give it to him or her. You should also investigate using moderated chat rooms. Moderators are there to keep an eye on the content and flow of chat conversation. They also have the authority to kick people who are misbehaving out of the chats. As with mailing lists, rules of common courtesy prevail in chat rooms. Do not harass others, do not flame, and avoid obscene and suggestive language.

Making Friends

If you chat regularly, you may begin to see familiar names and become friends with your fellow chatters. You may fall in love. You may meet someone and get married. I know people who have done all three. You also may find yourself in a difficult and potentially dangerous situation. As with anything in life, be careful and do not throw caution to the winds. The Internet, just like personal ads in the newspaper, has a dark side.

Remember that people can hide behind aliases on the Internet. A person can claim to be anyone or anything. Be careful with the personal information you divulge. If someone seems particularly aggressive or demanding, just stop talking. Get out of the room, or report the offender to the moderator. Many people ask for pictures, because it is fun to know what the person you are talking with looks like. But you do not have to share a picture if you do not want to. It is entirely your decision.

Be careful with "red flag" requests. Why would a stranger ask you for money? Or ask about intimate details of your home, your address, or phone number? Be cautious with the information you share. Do not be pressured into answering questions. Give friendships time to grow and develop naturally.

That said, I have met some great people on the Internet, and we have met in person and become good friends. The Internet is making our world smaller and giving all of us the opportunity to meet people we might never have met otherwise. But I used caution and common sense in allowing these friendships to develop.

INTERNET TELEPHONY

Once you have conquered mailing lists and chat rooms, your next step will probably be Internet telephony, which allows you to *talk* to friends, loved ones, or even total strangers. With just a microphone, computer, and the right software, it is possible to communicate verbally, long distance, for free, at least for now. Too good to be true? As with any emerging technology, glitches exist that need to be overcome before Web-based telephone service is as reliable as the standby telephone on the corner of your desk.

What exactly is Internet telephony, or VoIP, and how does it work? Basically, it is the two-way transmission of audio over an Internet protocol (IP) network. VoIP stands for "Voice over Internet protocol." Dazzle your friends at your next get-together by casually throwing "VoIP" into the conversation! Internet telephony allows calls to be made either from one computer to another, or from a computer to a telephone. In either case, calls are toll free or at least considerably less expensive than traditional telephone service, regardless if you are calling another city, state, or country.

VoIP is Internet based, so the signal is digital as compared with the traditional analog telephone. The digital signal is transmitted faster and in less space, which allows more calls to be transmitted over the line. This is the reason that many businesses are investigating VoIP as a way of handling larger call volume at much less cost.

But you are not a business, you are an individual, wondering if you can call your relatives overseas or children at college for free, right? If you are willing to put up with less-than-perfect reception and a bit of preplanning before your conversations, then yes, this is possible.

The first step is to make sure that you have the proper equipment. A computer with an Internet connection is required, along with a sound card, speakers, and microphone. You may opt for headphones with a microphone attached, but this is not essential. Next, you need the software to make the voice connection from one computer to another. A number of freeware and shareware programs are available. Each program has various bells and whistles, but most incorporate the capability for voice- or text-based conversation, and have features such as voice mail, messaging, telephone books, and call logs. Some programs include video capability so you can see the person with whom you are chatting, which, of course, requires a camera to record and transmit the image. You can download various programs from the Internet and give them a try to see which one suits you.

To make a call, the recipient requires a similar setup and needs to be using the same software. Unless the program has a voice mail option, both individuals need to arrange to be online at the same time and have the software up and running. The call is placed using an e-mail address (or IP address, if known). The telephone rings, the recipient answers, and voilà—conversation online.

Although setup of these programs is more or less automatic, each requires some tweaking. Typical problems include volume (microphone and speakers too soft or loud), calls breaking up, feedback, and an annoying tendency to be able to hear yourself speak through a several-second delay. Usually, these problems can be resolved by reading the Help file, visiting the online support site, or just playing with the various settings to get the right combination of call speed, volume, and sound.

CHAPTER 5

■■

A Guide to the Directory of Sites

The preceding four chapters have given you an overview of the Internet, an introduction to the tools necessary for exploration, and a summary of the sites you can expect to see. This chapter introduces you to the heart of the book: Part II, the Directory of Sites.

ABOUT THE DIRECTORY OF SITES

As you turn to the Directory of Sites, the first thing you will notice is that it is in alphabetical order. This has advantages and disadvantages. The advantage is that it facilitates finding something quickly; the disadvantage is that many sites have names that are not fully illustrative of the content included at the site. However, there is a detailed, cross-referenced index at the back of the book and I encourage you to turn to that if you are looking for something in particular. For example, Beth Rodgers' site, named "The Cave" (www.uwm.edu/People/brodg/), has some excellent links on philosophy, but you would not necessarily discern that from the name of the site. Using the index would provide this information. If you are looking for something in particular, make sure to check the index first to make the information in the Directory more accessible.

The next thing to notice is that each entry follows a similar format. A typical Directory entry is illustrated in Figure 5-1. The first line includes one of the following icons:

Type of site logo ☞   **Agency for Health Care Research**
Name of site ☞   **and Quality (AHRQ)**

Site address ☞   www.ahrq.gov

Site description ☞   The AHRQ (formerly the Agency for Health Care
                       Policy and Research) Website has links to its 14
                       offices and centers, news and resources, the
                       Research Activities online newsletter, data and
                       methods information, clinical practice
                       guidelines, available grants, an electronic
                       catalog, a search function, and other useful
                       resources. They are regularly adding many new
                       features. The site includes a link to the
                       Department of Health and Human Services. The
                       AHRQ list is available by sending an e-mail to
                       listserv@list.ahrq.gov (type subscribe in the
                       subject line and sub public_list-L Firstname
                       Lastname in the body of the message. This list
                       runs on the Listserv program; you will receive a
                       reply to confirm your intention to join the list.

Contact information ☞   Contact: info@ahrq.gov

FIGURE 5-1. Sample entry in the Directory of Sites.

 means it is a site on the World Wide Web (WWW);

 refers to Listserv mailing list groups; and

 refers to Usenet news groups.

There are very few U sites; the majority that are listed are from the WWW or are mailing lists (L).

Following the site icon is the name of the site. This name is taken directly from the name present at the site. I have not changed names from those given by the developers. All sites in the Directory are arranged in strict alphabetical order (with the exception of the word "The," which has either been deleted or the site is alphabetized by the first word after "The"). Thus, Bo Graham's home page is under B; The American Association of Nurse Anesthetists is under A; and NursingCenter.com (where you can find information on *Computers in Nursing*) is under N. My colleague, Susan Newbold, was upset when she thought her home page was excluded from the first edition, because she wasn't listed under S or N. She found herself under H, because she has named her page "Home Page of Susan K. Newbold." Through three editions of this book, she has not renamed her site, so she is still in the "aitches" (H).

Following the name of the site is the address. Once again, this item has been taken directly from the site. For sites that have multiple pages, I have included the address of the home page or first page of the site. For mailing lists, I have included the address to which you send your message to subscribe. I have also included the software on which the list is running (LISTSERV, LISTPROC, and so on) and whether you will be asked to confirm your intention to subscribe to the list. I did not include the address of the list where you send your message to post to the group. That information will be sent to you once you are subscribed successfully to a group. A description of the typical process for subscribing, unsubscribing, and managing your subscription is included in detail in Chapter 3. A summary of mailing list commands is also included in Chapter 3; using the information in that chapter along with the information included in the Directory should be all you need to become successfully subscribed to a mailing list of interest.

Next is a brief description of the site. In many cases, I have used the descriptions provided by the sites themselves, embellishing when necessary. If a site has a particularly useful or unusual feature, I have included that information. Unusual features are often the keys to how the site is cross-referenced in the Index. If the site includes specific contact information, I have included that information, which may be a person's name and e-mail address or just an e-mail address. Note that I have not included mailing addresses, phone numbers, or fax numbers, although that information might be available at the site. Because this is a guide to the Internet, I chose to include Internet contact information exclusively.

ABOUT THE INDEX

As mentioned earlier, the index is a detailed, cross-referenced listing of sites and text in the first part of the book. With respect to the sites, I have discovered in my Internet travels that the name of a page or a site is not always descriptive of the content that is included. For example, Bo Graham has put together an excellent page of nursing, medical, and health resources (http://bgraham.com/nursing/). It has many useful links, including several for oncology and cancer-related information. A name like "Bo Graham's Home Page" unfortunately does not provide an inkling of what is included in the page. But a quick check under "cancer" in the Index would point you to Bo's Website.

HOW SITES WERE SELECTED

When I put together the first edition of this book with my friend and colleague Teena Ouellette, we faced a daunting task. There are millions of URLs on the World Wide Web alone, plus telnet sites, FTP, mailing lists, and Usenet discussion groups. The situation has only become more overwhelming through the second and now third editions of the book. At last count, some estimate that there are over 14 million Websites presently available on the Internet, and that number is increasing daily! To decide what to include in the Directory, I needed to develop some explicit criteria to evaluate sites. The following guidelines have been used through all three editions of this book and have served me well in each instance.

First, this book is designed as a guide, not an encyclopedia. I have tried to be selective; my goal was not to include every site that had something to do with nursing and health but to select sites that clearly provided useful information or, in some cases, links to other sites. If you are working in a particular specialty area, once you become comfortable with Internet exploring, I am sure that you will find sites related to your area of interest and expertise that are not included in this guide. Even so, I hope that the sites that are included set you on the right path on your journey and ultimately point you to more specialized sites of interest. Remember my earlier suggestion to take advantage of links!

I tried to include one, two, or three sites on a wide variety of topics, but I did not try to be exhaustive on any particular topic. Use these sites as a suggestion or a starting point, and then begin your own exploration. My approach in selecting sites for the Directory was to favor quality over quantity.

I looked at the date when a site was last updated to determine whether or not to include it. Generally, I wanted evidence that the site was being regularly maintained and updated. Dates needed to be in within the last 18 months to be included. With the rapid changes in health care and nursing, I figured that if a site developer has not updated a site for more than 18 months, that called into question the accuracy of the information included. The cut-off date was somewhat arbitrary, but I found it worked well to evaluate sites.

I tried to assess whether or not a site was a "going concern" in making the decision whether or not to include it. Schools of nursing and associations are obviously not going to disappear overnight. On the other hand, there are many individual home pages that just do not look like they are going to be around for the long haul. If I got repeated error messages in trying to visit a site or had problems with connection on an ongoing basis, that increased the likelihood that a site was not included.

I assessed sites for the usefulness of their content. Sites that are nothing more than a series of links to other sites ranked lower on my selection list, unless the links were very unusual or particularly comprehensive. Sites that included good content, as well as links, were deemed to be useful and included in the guide.

I also evaluated the credentials of the people involved with the site and their clarity in communicating that message to others. For example, the OCD Home

Page (http://fairlite.com/ocd/) is a site developed by a man with obsessive-compulsive disorder and his wife. He is very clear that he is not a medical or health professional and that the information offered at the site is not a substitute for medical treatment and care. Even so, I found the site to be of great interest and contained many useful resources; thus, I opted to include it.

I looked for a way to contact the site developers, either through e-mail or a feedback page. Site developers that are "anonymous"—that is, not encouraging feedback or being forthcoming about their credentials—did not make it into the book.

I also kept in mind the criteria for evaluation from the Health on the Net Foundation (see Chapter 3 for a more thorough discussion). Sites that were blatantly commercial and existed only to sell a product were not included. Sites where the developer put him or herself forth as the "worldwide leading expert" on a particular topic, but had no evidence to support the claim (e.g., publications included in a MEDLINE search) were not included. If I had any questions about the true intentions of the site developer or if there were any ethical concerns on my part, I erred on the side of caution and did not include the URL.

WHAT IS NOT INCLUDED

Taking the quality, not quantity approach to selection, there are some useful resources that are not included in the Directory but are still available to you on the Web. The following types of sites were not included, or included in a selective manner.

Libraries

I opted not to include a listing of the many health and science libraries that are available via telnet. In my experience, most people connect to their local or regional library for card catalog searching. For more extensive resources, I recommend the National Library of Medicine, which is included in the Directory. If you have need to search a specific health science library, you can generally connect to it from the associated university home page. To find these libraries, try brute force: www.nameofuniversity.edu. The name of the university might be an abbreviation (UNH) or the full name (Washington, for the University of Washington). Once you connect to the university, find the link to the library.

Hospitals

Like libraries, there are many hospital sites on the Web. Many of these sites would be useful for patients seeking care or nurses seeking employment: they have lists of staff, phone numbers, parking information, job postings, and the like. I chose not to include these many listings. If you are interested in finding a particular hos-

pital, a good starting place is HospitalWeb (http://neuro-www.mgh.harvard.
edu/hospitalweb.shtml), which has a constantly growing list of hospital Websites
from around the country.

Schools of Nursing

When I wrote the first edition of this book, I included about 53 sites for Schools
and Colleges of Nursing. That was pretty much the universe of nursing school
and college Websites at that time. Since then, there has been an explosion of sites.
Many of them, however, are nothing more than the catalog put online. Although
that might be a very useful resource to current and prospective students, I did not
think that it would be terribly helpful for my readers. Thus, I have included only
those school and college Websites that had something above and beyond the program description and faculty roster. I have identified these extras in the Directory.

If you are interested in finding a particular school or college to learn more
about the program, visit Nursing-HealthWeb (http://www.lib.umich.edu/
hw/nursing.html). This site has a comprehensive lists of nursing programs. And
if the program you want is not on one of those lists, try brute force—it really
works!

Government Listings

Although I included many federal government agencies, I did not include listings
of each state government Website, nor did I include listing for the House of Rep-
resentatives and the Senate. A good list can be found at AORN Online
(http://www.aorn.org) in the legislative section.

The Personal Touch

To select sites, I visited each and every Website listed in the Directory, some several times. I subscribed to every mailing list included to verify the address and
purpose. For the descriptions, I relied on what the list returned to me as an introduction. If you subscribe and the discussion is not what you expected, it is easy
enough to unsubscribe.

Finally, I tried as much as possible to be objective, but this Internet business is
fraught with subjectivity. My personal biases and areas of interest will probably
show through here and there in sites and descriptions, but my goal was to be as
broad based as possible. My experience in nursing, public policy, and management, as well as my experience serving as Editor-in-Chief of *Computers in Nursing*,
contributed to the overall selection process.

To this end, I would appreciate your feedback. If there are particular sites you
like that I have not included, please send me the information. Many of the sites
included in this third edition came directly from readers' suggestions. My e-mail
address is LeslieN@usm.maine.edu or LNICOLL@maine.rr.com. There are are
also links to my address at the *Computers in Nursing* home page (go to the journals

section of NursingCenter.com) for you to communicate with me directly. If there is a site that you feel would be a useful addition to this book, send it to me, along with the complete address and a brief description. Similarly, if there are sites that are included that are no longer active or just not useful, please let me know that, too. I consider this guide to be a work in progress and will be updating it with information that I receive from readers. I look forward to hearing from you.

As I noted earlier, an informed traveler is an intelligent traveler. Take a few minutes to familiarize yourself with the information contained in the Directory. And then, you'll be ready to begin your journey.

PART II

DIRECTORY OF SITES

AANURSES

AANURSES@ontosystems.com

Discussion group for nurses and other healthcare professionals in recovery from alcoholism, drug addiction, eating disorders, gambling, codependency, and obsessive-compulsive disease. This list is confidential, and requests to join are screened by the list owner.

Subscribe

 Aboriginal Nurses Association of Canada

www.anac.on.ca

Welcome to the Aboriginal Nurses Association of Canada online! ANAC is a nongovernmental, nonprofit organization striving for better health for the Indian and Inuit people. An affiliate group of the Canadian Nurses Association, it is the only Aboriginal professional nursing organization in Canada.

Contact: info@anac.on.ca

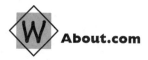 **About.com**

www.about.com

If you need information on a topic but have no idea where to begin, consider visiting about.com. This smorgasbord of sites, links, and information has entries on hundreds of topics, each led by "expert guides" who cull the information and post articles, links, and resources. In their words "About.com one of the best places to go to know more about, well, anything." There are sites for nursing, health issues, diseases, patient education, consumer education, and more.

ACOR—Association of Cancer Online Resources

www.acor.org

ACOR is a starting point for a variety of online resources related to cancer. A particularly useful feature is the list archives, a searchable database of most of the existing cancer-related news lists on the Internet. The archives is a "living medical encyclopedia" wherein visitors can search the archives and indexes of cancer Listservs covering brain, hematologic, breast, ovarian, and prostate cancer. ACOR also hosts a growing number of cancer resource sites by patients, their supporters, and organizations.

 ADDCTNSG

Listproc@list.ab.umd.edu

Discussion list for the scholarly, academic, and clinical issues related to the practice of addictions nursing. The list runs on the Listproc system. On subscribing, you will be asked to confirm your intention of joining the list.

Subscribe ADDCTNSG Firstname Lastname

 ADDULT

listserv@maelstrom.stjohns.edu

Discussion group for adults with attention-deficit disorder. Runs on the Listserv program. When your request to join is confirmed, you will be asked to send an e-mail to the list owner introducing yourself.

Subscribe ADDULT Firstname Lastname

 Adopt-A-Greyhound

www.adopt-a-greyhound.org

Website of The Greyhound Project, Inc., with information on greyhound adoption and rescue. Good resources for greyhounds as family pets.

Agency for Health Care Research and Quality (AHRQ)

www.ahrq.gov

The AHRQ (formerly the Agency for Health Care Policy and Research) Website has links to its 14 offices and centers, news and resources, the Research Activities online newsletter, data and methods information, clinical practice guidelines, available grants, an electronic catalog, a search function, and other useful resources. They are regularly adding many new features. The site includes a link to the Department of Health and Human Services. The AHRQ list is available by sending an e-mail to listserv@list.ahrq.gov (type subscribe in the subject line and sub public_list-L Firstname Lastname in the body of the message). This list runs on the Listserv program; you will receive a reply to confirm your intention to join the list.

Contact: info@ahrq.gov

 AGING-DD

listserv@ukcc.uky.edu

Aging-DD is an open forum that welcomes discussion, information, and materials on aging and older persons with developmental disabilities. This list runs on the Listserv program; you will receive a reply to confirm your intention to join the list.

Subscribe AGING-DD Firstname Lastname

 AIDS Clinical Trials

www.critpath.org/trials.htm

This site features the full texts of open protocols of the major clinical trials networks. You may also peruse guides to entering clinical trials and evaluating them, expanded access programs, buyers' clubs, and patient assistance programs.

Contact: kiyoshi@critpath.org

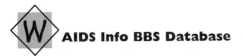

AIDS Info BBS Database

http://aidsinfobbs.org

Here is a treasure-house of information about AIDS. It has been building since 1985, always selecting the best but never accumulating the most. You will find that much of your selection work has already been done for you before you begin reading here. On controversial points, this collection presents both sides of the major issues, clearly labeled so you can avoid them if desired.

Contact: Ben Gardiner, ben@aidsinfobbs.org

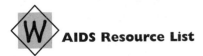

AIDS Resource List

www.specialweb.com/aids/

This page offers annotated links to AIDS-related Websites, Gophers, and Usenets throughout the world. Visitors here are also invited to show support for preventing the spread of HIV and for those with the disease by downloading a small red ribbon from this Website and placing it on their own Web pages.

Contact: aids@specialweb.com

ALLERGY

Listserv@listserv.uark.edu

A discussion group on allergies, for allergy sufferers, and health professionals. The list runs on the Listserv system. On subscribing, you will be asked to confirm your intention of joining the list.

Subscribe ALLERGY Firstname Lastname

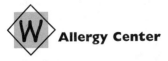

Allergy Center

www.onlineallergycenter.com

In 1995, the On-Line Allergy Center was established by Russell Roby, JD, MD, to provide helpful allergy tips and information to allergy sufferers worldwide. This Website has no sponsors and offers all information as a public service.

Contact: allergy@allergy-center.com

Allergy Internet Resources–AIR

www.immune.com/allergy/allabc.html

An index to documents and sites on the Internet with information about allergies of all kinds. The index is divided into the following categories: General Information; Asthma; Food Allergies; Kids' Allergies; Latex Allergy; Hay Fever, Airborne, and Seasonal Allergies; Skin Allergies; and Stings, Testing, and Anaphylaxis. A link at the bottom of the index will take you to information about the allergy e-mail discussion group, complete with an archive of recent postings to the group.

Contact: Allergylinks@immune.com

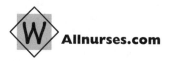 **Alliance of Genetic Support Groups**

www.geneticalliance.org

The Genetic Alliance (formerly The Alliance of Genetic Support Groups, Inc.), is an international coalition of individuals, professionals, and genetic support organizations working together to enhance the lives of everyone impacted by genetic conditions.

Contact: info@geneticalliance.org

 Allnurses.com

www.allnurses.com

Formerly Worldwide Nurse, Allnurses.com is developed and maintained by Brian Short, RN. This Website hosts nursing bulletin boards and has pointers to other nursing resources, disease links, search forms, and medical software reviews.

Contact: webmaster@allnurses.com

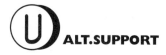 **ALT.SUPPORT**

The Usenet groups that start with "alt.support" tend to be discussions among patients, families, and interested persons, including health professionals, about diseases, health problems, disabilities, and the like. Some of the alt.support Usenet groups cover abortion, AIDS, arthritis, asthma, breastfeeding, cancer, cerebral palsy, chronic pain, depression, diabetes, endometriosis, epilepsy, glau-coma, hemophilia, herpes, menopause, multiple sclerosis, obsessive-compulsive disorder, ostomy, post-polio syndrome, schizophrenia, sleep disorders, thyroid disease, tinnitus, and post-traumatic stress disorder.

 Alternative Medicine Home Page

www.pitt.edu/~cbw/altm.html

Maintained by the Falk Library for the Health Sciences at the University of Pitts-burgh, this page is a jump station for sources of information on unconventional, unorthodox, unproven, or alternative, complementary, innovative, integrative therapies.

Contact: Charles B. Wessel, cbw+@pitt.edu

 Alzheimer Research Forum

www.alzforum.org

The Alzheimer Research Forum is a nonprofit foundation that established this Website to serve the scientific and clinical research community. The site also pro-vides information for family members and caregivers. Handy references to other Websites of interest to this community include postings for job openings, jobs sought, and research collaborations, as well as links to major Websites for job advertisements in the life sciences; listings of upcoming meetings; links to rele-vant research centers with their own Websites; a list of Website links; and a directory to online journals in the fields of Alzheimer's disease, neurology, and neuroscience.

 Alzheimer's Association

www.alz.org

Visitors can find the Alzheimer's Association mission statement here, as well as facts about Alzheimer's disease, a recent archive of media releases, and position statements. Medical researchers interested in funding for research on Alzheimer's disease will find information about research grant programs. There is also a listing of 200 chapter locations, caregiver resources, medical informa-tion, conferences and events, and links to other Alzheimer's Web pages.

Contact: info@alz.org

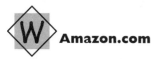 **Amazon.com**

www.amazon.com

"Earth's Biggest Selection" with 2.5 million books plus auctions, home improvement, electronics, and toys. Secure online ordering and speedy delivery. You can buy nursing books here, many at a discount.

 American Academy of Child and Adolescent Psychiatry (AACAP)

www.aacap.org

Website of the AACAP. The legislative tracking service is a new addition. A particularly useful component of this page is a collection of 73 ``Facts for Families,'' fact sheets on various problems of childhood and adolescence. The sheets are available in English, French, and Spanish, and may be downloaded, copied, and distributed as needed.

Contact: postmaster@aacap.org

 American Academy of Pain Management (AAPM)

www.aapainmanage.org

Website of the American Academy of Pain Management (AAPM). AAPM is the largest multidisciplinary pain society and the largest physician-based pain society in the United States. The site includes information on the organization and membership, and a variety of patient resources. It is also possible to access the National Pain Databank, with live data on treatments and outcomes for specific conditions, and a new Research Assistant computer program to research specific conditions.

Contact: aapm@aapainmanage.org

American Academy of Pediatrics (AAP)

www.aap.org

A voice for children for more than 70 years, the American Academy of Pediatrics (AAP) is an organization of 55,000 pediatricians dedicated to the health, safety, and well-being of infants, children, adolescents, and young adults. The AAP Website has news, a press release archive, membership information, child health resources, and information for parents and health professionals. Secure ordering of AAP products is available through their online bookstore.

Contact: kidsdocs@aap.org or webmaster@aap.org

 American Association for the History of Nursing (AAHN)

www.aahn.org

The American Association for the History of Nursing (AAHN) is a professional organization open to everyone interested in the history of nursing. Originally founded in 1978 as a historical methodology group, the association was briefly named the International History of Nursing Society. The organization's purposes are to foster the importance of history as relevant to understanding the past, defining the present, and influencing the future of nursing by stimulating national and international interest and collaboration in the history of nursing; educating nurses and the public regarding the history and heritage of the nursing profession; encouraging and supporting research in the history of nursing and recognizing outstanding scholarly achievement in nursing history; encouraging the collection, preservation, and use of materials of historical importance to nursing; serving as a resource for information about nursing history; producing and distributing educational materials related to the history and heritage of the nursing profession; promoting the inclusion of nursing history in nursing curricula; and fostering interdisciplinary collaboration in history.

Contact: aahn@ahhn.org

 American Association for Therapeutic Humor

www.aath.org

Working at a frenzied pace in a hospital or doctor's office would be enough to wear down anyone's funny bone. As a counterbalance, the American Association for Therapeutic Humor was created to help health professionals maintain a sense of humor about the world around them. The AATH Website features a collection of articles from the therapeutic humor literature, plus a collection of "Twelve Affirmations of Positive Humor" and links to other therapeutic humor Websites.

Contact: office@aath.org

 American Association of Colleges of Nursing

www.aacn.nche.edu

Website of AACN, the national voice for America's baccalaureate- and higher-degree nursing education programs.

Contact: webmaster@aacn.nche.edu

 American Association of Critical-Care Nurses

www.aacn.org

The American Association of Critical-Care Nurses was founded in 1969 and now, 31 years later, has grown to become the world's largest specialty nursing organization. The vision of AACN is a healthcare system, driven by the needs of patients, in which critical care nurses make their optimal contribution. This searchable site has full-text journal articles, information on certification, publications, and public policy, as well as an online catalog, a list of association chapters, and membership information.

Contact: info@aacn.org

 American Association of Diabetes Educators (AADE)

www.aadenet.org

AADE is made up of a wide variety of health professionals who are involved in educating people with diabetes. AADE has a number of state and regional chapters, puts on educational conferences for health professionals, and is a great source (via the Diabetes Educator Access Line) for referrals to nurse educators and physicians in your area who specialize in diabetes. The organization sponsors the C.D.E. certification program for diabetes educators. It also provides some grants, scholarships, and awards for educational research and teaching activities.

Contact: aade@aadenet.org

American Association of Legal Nurse Consultants

www.aalnc.org

The American Association of Legal Nurse Consultants (AALNC) is a nonprofit organization dedicated to the professional enhancement of registered nurses practicing in a consulting capacity in the legal field. Founded in 1989, AALNC serves as a resource for its members by providing opportunities for continuing education and an exchange of information on matters relating to legal nurse consulting, medical care, and healthcare law.

Contact: info@aalnc.org

 American Association of Neuroscience Nurses (AANN)

www.aann.org

Founded in 1968, the American Association of Neuroscience Nurses is a national organization of 3,400 registered nurses and other healthcare professionals dedicated to improving the care of the neuroscience patient and to furthering the interests of health professionals in the neurosciences. AANN's membership represents nurses and healthcare professionals working in diverse areas of neuroscience: multispecialty and neuroscience intensive care units. The Website contains information about the association and links to neuroscience nursing resources.

Contact: aann@aann.org

 American Association of Nurse Anesthetists (AANA)

www.aana.com

The AANA Website features news, events, and professional and patient resources. Patients can access related information describing anesthesia and its affects and their role in the recovery process. Members can find organizational information such as contacts, events, educational offerings, and anesthesia-related Web resources. Professional resources include information on history, legal issues, cost-effectiveness of nurse anesthesia practice, and educational opportunities.

Contact: info@aana.com

American Association of Occupational Health Nurses

www.aaohn.org

This is the Website of the AAOHN, whose mission is to advance the profession of occupational and environmental health nursing. News, practice resources, and a discussion forum are among the offerings featured on the site.

Contact: e-mail directly from the site

 American Cancer Society

www.cancer.org

The American Cancer Society Website has information on their organization and local chapters, press releases, extensive information on cancer prevention and treatment, a calendar of events, publications, and resources. There are also pointers to the Relay for Life, Making Strides, and Cars for a Cure.

Contact: e-mail directly from the site

 American College of Nurse Midwives (ACNM)

www.acnm.org

The mission of ACNM is to promote the health and well-being of women and infants within their families and communities through the development and support of the profession of midwifery as practiced by certified nurse-midwives and certified midwives. The philosophy inherent in the profession states that nurse-midwives believe every individual has the right to safe, satisfying health care with respect for human dignity and cultural variations. The ACNM site has information on how to find nurse-midwives, nurse-midwifery education and certification, ACNM and professional information, ACNM chapter information, press releases, and other nursing resources.

Contact: info@acnm.org

American College of Nurse Practitioners

www.nurse.org/acnp/

Website of the American College of Nurse Practitioners. Founded in 1993, the ACNP is a national nonprofit membership organization headquartered in Washington, DC. The ACNP is focused on advocacy and keeping nurse practitioners current on legislative, regulatory and clinical practice issues that effect them in the rapidly changing healthcare arena.

Contact: acnp@nurse.org

 American Diabetes Association

www.diabetes.org

The mission of the American Diabetes Association is to prevent and cure diabetes, and to improve the lives of all people affected by diabetes. To fulfill this mission, the American Diabetes Association funds research; publishes scientific findings; and provides information and other services to people with diabetes, their families, healthcare professionals, and the public. This Website has the latest news on diabetes, an information directory, full-text journal articles, and on online store. Visitors can also find contact information for local offices.

Contact: webmaster@diabetes.org

 American Forensic Nurses

www.amrn.com

Information on American Forensic Nurses, their work, and their goals. Distance courses that can be taken through the WWW are available at this site, providing registered nurses interested in the field of forensic sciences specialized educational programs and training conferences.

Contact: e-mail directly from the site

American Heart Association (AHA)

www.americanheart.org

The American Heart Association Web page contains information about the organization, patient information, support group links, licensed products and services, and science and research. There are also pointers to other heart and cardiovascular servers maintained by government agencies and nongovernment societies and associations. An excellent patient-oriented area, Living with Heart Failure, can be found at www.americanheart.org/chf/.

Contact: e-mail directly from the site

 American Holistic Nurses' Association

www.ahna.org

Website of the AHNA, this site contains information on the association, education, certification, and standards for holistic nursing. The goal of the American Holistic Nurses' Association is to bring concepts of holism to all areas of nursing practice. Since 1981, AHNA members have worked to integrate holistic principles into their own lives, as well as into nursing, education, clinical practice and nursing research.

Contact: ahna-flag@flaglink.com

 American Liver Foundation

www.liverfoundation.org

Website of the American Liver Foundation, the only national, voluntary non-profit health agency dedicated to preventing, treating, and curing hepatitis and all liver diseases through research, education, and support groups. Site includes information for physicians, nurses, other health professionals, patients, and their families.

Contact: webmail@liverfoundation.org

American Lung Association

www.lungusa.org

"When you can't breathe, nothing else matters." The American Lung Association (ALA) is the oldest voluntary health organization in the United States, with a national office and constituent and affiliate associations around the country. Founded in 1904 to fight tuberculosis, ALA today fights lung disease in all its forms, with special emphasis on asthma, tobacco control, and environmental health.

Contact: webmaster@lungusa.org

 American Medical Association

www.ama-assn.org

Website of the AMA. This searchable site includes full text of selected articles from their journals, including *JAMA*, news releases, and abstracts. There are information centers on migraine, asthma, HIV/AIDS, and women's health. The On-Line Doctor Finder is a handy resource for patients and professionals.

Contact: e-mail directly from the site

 American Nurses Association

www.ana.org or www.nursingworld.org

Website of the ANA with links to state organizations, legislative issues, and membership information. This site is also the home of the American Academy of Nursing, American Nurses Credentialing Center, and the American Nurses Foundation. Access The American Nurse, classified advertising, and legislative information. Links to state nursing associations are also available. The Online Journal of Issues in Nursing (see separate listing for OJIN) can be accessed via this site.

Contact: webmaster@ana.org

American Physiological Society

www.faseb.org/aps/

The American Physiological Society is devoted to fostering scientific research, education, and the dissemination of scientific information. By providing a spectrum of physiological information, the Society strives to play a role in the progress of science and the advancement of knowledge. Providing current, usable information to the physiological community is the Society's primary focus.

Contact: webmaster@aps.faseb.org

 American Public Health Association

www.apha.org

The American Public Health Association (APHA) is the oldest and largest organization of public health professionals in the world, representing more than 50,000 members from over 50 occupations of public health. APHA's Website includes information on its programs and projects, legislative issues, publications, and state associations.

Contact: comments@apha.org

 American Red Cross

www.redcross.org

A public relations platform for the American Red Cross, this site is maintained by the national headquarters. The mission, goals, history, financial structure, and health and safety programs of the national arm of this humanitarian organization are fully detailed. Of particular interest are the current press releases that detail relief efforts in disaster areas. The Virtual Museum takes you on an ever-changing voyage through the diverse cultural history of the Red Cross.

Contact: internet@usa.redcross.org

American Society of PeriAnesthesia Nurses

www.aspan.org

Here is the Website of ASPAN, with membership information and resources relating to perianesthesia nursing.

Contact: aspan@slackinc.com

 Americans With Disabilities Act Document Center

http://janweb.icdi.wvu.edu/kinder/

This Website contains copies of the Americans With Disabilities Act of 1990 (ADA), ADA regulations, technical assistance manuals prepared by the United States Equal Employment Opportunity Commission (EEOC) or the United States Department of Justice (DOJ), and other technical assistance documents sponsored by the National Institute on Disability and Rehabilitation Research (NIDRR) and reviewed by EEOC or DOJ. There are also links to other Internet sources of information concerning disability issues, legal issues, occupational health and safety, and total quality management issues. Visitors searching for an item not found on this site can use the Internet search tools and links to libraries that this site provides. Visitors can also find information and links for the Job Accommodation Network (JAN).

Contact: Duncan Kinder, dckinder@mountain.net

 AMIA Nursing Informatics Working Group

www.amia-niwg.org

The overall goal of AMIA's Nursing Informatics Working Group is to promote the advancement of nursing informatics within the larger multidisciplinary context of health informatics. The organization and its members pursue this goal in many arenas: professional practice, education, research, governmental and other service, professional organizations, and industry.

Contact: webdiva@amia-niwg.org

AMPUTEE

listserv@sjuvm.stjohns.edu

Discussion group for amputees, friends, families, and health professionals. The list runs on the Listserv system. Requests to join are forwarded to the list owner for approval.

Subscribe AMPUTEE Firstname Lastname

 An American Nurse at War

www.nurse-at-war.org

An American Nurse at War is a video documentary. This Website mirrors the film and is designed as an additional learning resource about World War I history and early twentieth century women's history. Red Cross nurse Marion McCune Rice cared for wounded soldiers in France during World War I. The Website offers a virtual classroom around that experience, including a curriculum guide, stories of Red Cross nurses, and a collection of Marion McCune's letters, as well as more than 60 historic photographs.

Contact: shoop@cheshire.net

 ANEST-L

listserv@listserv.acsu.buffalo.edu

Discussion group for anesthesiologists, nurse anesthetists, and others interested in anesthesiology and critical care. This list runs on the Listserv system. You will receive a reply requesting confirmation of your intention to join the list.

Subscribe ANEST-L Firstname Lastname

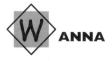 **ANNA**

http://anna.inurse.com

Official Website of the American Nephrology Nurses Association.

Contact: webmaster@inurse.com

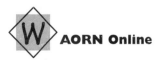 **AORN Online**

www.aorn.org

Visitors to AORN Online can obtain information on the Association of periOperative Registered Nurses, Inc. (AORN) and its activities. New features include a search function from every page, an expansive help section, and a new bookstore. There are pointers to organizational information, products and services, clinical practice information, education, government affairs, online perioperative employment opportunities, certification, and industry connections. This site also includes the "Surgery Center: A Patient's Place," a resource of patient-centered information specifically relating to surgery and the surgical process. There is a feedback form for visitor input and general membership information for AORN.

Contact: Website@aorn.org

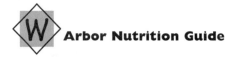 **Arbor Nutrition Guide**

www.arborcom.com

A site of more than 1,000 nutrition resources. Easily searchable and well organized.

Contact: update@arborcom.com

 Arkansas State University College of Nursing and Health Professions

www.astate.edu/docs/acad/conhp/hp/dean.htm

This site has information on the College of Nursing and its programs. There is a useful link to the Delta Health Education Partnership from this site.

Contact: slesh@crow.astate.edu

ARL E-JOURNAL

Listproc@arl.org

Maintained by the Association of Research Libraries, this site is a discussion list on electronic journals (e-journals). This list runs on the Listproc system. You will be automatically subscribed to the list when a request is submitted to join.

Subscribe ARL-EJOURNAL Firstname Lastname.

 Arthritis Foundation

www.arthritis.org

The mission of the Arthritis Foundation is to support research to find the cure for and prevention of arthritis, and to improve the quality of life for those affected by arthritis. Visitors to the Arthritis Foundation Web page will find news updates, fact sheets, research resources, and chapter locations. There are also links to other organizations devoted to fighting arthritis in adults and children.

Contact: webmaster@arthritis.org

 Association of Rehabilitation Nurses

www.rehabnurse.org

Website for the ARN. The site includes an online forum, membership information; continuing education opportunities; news; periodicals; information on certification, grants, and scholarships; and general information for the public.

Contact: info@rehabnurse.org

 Association of Women's Health, Obstetric and Neonatal Nursing

www.awhonn.org

Official Website of AWHONN, whose mission is to promote excellence in nursing practice to improve the health of women and newborns. This site provides information on the organization and a wide variety of resources for obstetric, neonatal, and women's health care.

Contact: janac@awhonn.org

 Australian Electronic Journal of Nursing Education

www.scu.edu.au/schools/nhcp/aejne/aejnehpa.htm

The *AEJNE* is committed to enhancing the teaching and learning experience across a variety of nurse contexts. The journal is a means by which nurses can share findings, insights, experience, and advice with colleagues involved in all aspects of the educational process. The *AEJNE* seeks to use the advantages of electronic communication to provide rapid and accessible information about teaching and learning to nurses worldwide. The *AEJNE* has a special commitment to nursing education in Australia. To this end, it will allow country-specific comment in this context. The universality of teaching and learning will, however, provide wide opportunity for nurses outside Australia to publish studies and papers in the journal.

Contact: aejne@scu.edu.au

 Autism Network International

www.ani.ac or www.staff.uiuc.edu/~bordner/ani/

Autism International Network International is an autistic-run self-help and advocacy organization for autistic people.

Contact: Jim Sinclair, jisincla@mailbox.syr.edu

 Ball State University School of Nursing

www.bsu.edu/nursing

This school of nursing's Website allows the visitor to access general information, academic program and course information, and distance education opportunities and to take a virtual tour of the Health Care Learning Resource Center.

Contact: Kay Hodson, khodson@bsu.edu

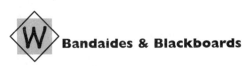

Bandaides & Blackboards

http://funrsc.fairfield.edu/~jfleitas/contents.html

This is a site about growing up with medical problems. Its goal is to help people understand what it's like from the perspective of the children and teens who are doing just that. These kids have become experts at coping with problems that most children have never heard of. They'd like you to know how they do it, and they hope that you'll be glad you came to visit. The site is divided into three areas: one for kids, one for teens, and one for adults. Lots of useful information and some moving stories and poems can be found here.

Contact: Joan Fleitas, fleitas@fair1.fairfield.edu

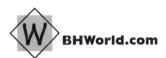

Best Practice Network

www.best4health.com or ww1.best4health.org/startbp.cfm

The purpose of the Best Practice Network is to promote information sharing in healthcare by nurses, physicians, and other healthcare professionals. The Best Practice Network facilitates the exchange of ideas, encourages collaboration in results-oriented problem solving, and enables healthcare professionals to share best practices and other creative solutions that will positively impact patient care and community well-being. The predominant goal is to develop realistic and sustainable healthcare initiatives that promote optimal patient care and have immediate and system-wide impact.

Contact: join-us@best4health.org

BHWorld.com

www.bhworld.com

BHWorld.com is an online service that is designed and developed exclusively for the behavioral health professional and clients/patients. The site encourages fellowship and sharing of experiences.

Contact: webmaster@essexconsulting.com

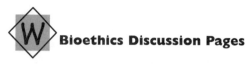 **Bioethics Discussion Pages**

www-hsc.usc.edu/~mbernste/index.html

This site includes ongoing discussions on a variety of ethical issues. Everyone is invited to join in the discussion regarding these issues. Current topics include patient quality of life, rights of insurance companies to generic test results, and social worth in the allocation of scarce resources.

Contact: Maurice Bernstein, MD, DoktorMo@aol.com

 Bioethics Online Service

www.mcw.edu/bioethics/bos.html

The Bioethics Online Service is a searchable database of abstracts of pertinent bioethics journal articles, legislative actions, and court decisions. It is maintained by the Center for the Study of Bioethics and the Office of Research, Technology, and Information of the Medical College of Wisconsin. The database is updated weekly.

Contact: Arthur R. Derse, aderse@its.mcw.edu

 BLIND-L

listserv@uafsysb.uark.edu

Discussion group about blindness and related issues. The list runs on the Listserv system. Upon subscribing, you will be asked to confirm your intention to join the list.

Subscribe BLIND-L Firstname Lastname

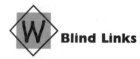 **Blind Links**

www.seidata.com/~marriage/rblind.html

A large collection of links to Internet sites related to blindness, compiled by Ron Marriage. Resources listed include adaptive technology, advocacy and training, books and magazines, commercial employment, medical links, mobility and Braille, U.S. Government links, and Websites of blind U.S. veterans.

Contact: Ron Marriage, marriage@seidata.com

BMT TALK

listserv@listserv.acor.org

Discussion group about bone marrow transplant and related issues. The list runs on the Listserv system. On subscribing, you will be asked to confirm your intention to join the list.

Subscribe BMT-TALK Firstname Lastname

 The Body: AIDS and HIV Information Resource

www.thebody.com

A remarkably comprehensive resource devoted to the myriad facets of the AIDS epidemic, including information on the disease, safe sex, support groups, treatment, mental health, and legal and financial issues. Materials published at the site come from a variety of governmental and private organizations.

 Bo Graham's Home Page

www.bgraham.com/nursing/

Bo Graham's pioneering Website. Although it is primarily a links page, there are many useful connections, especially related to cancer.

Contact: Bo Graham, bgraham@bgraham.com

 Boston College School of Nursing

www.bc.edu/bc_org/avp/son/

A stop here offers information on the undergraduate, master's, and doctoral programs; faculty; and scholarships. There are also links to the Center for Nursing Research, continuing education programs, Alpha Chi chapter of Sigma Theta Tau, and other nursing Websites.

Contact: donelan@bc.edu

BRAINTMR

listserv@mitvma.mit.edu

Discussion group for brain tumor patients, their families, and health professionals. The list runs on the Listserv system. Upon subscribing, you will be asked to confirm your intention to join the list.

Subscribe BRAINTMR Firstname Lastname

 BREAST-CANCER

listserv@morgan.ucs.mun.ca

Discussion group on breast cancer for patients, families, and health professionals. The list runs on the Listserv system. On subscribing, you will be asked to confirm your intention to join the list.

Subscribe BREAST-CANCER Firstname Lastname

 California Nurses' Association

www.calnurse.org

The purpose of the CNA is to foster high standards of nursing practice, to promote the professional and educational advancement of nurses, and to promote the welfare of nurses to the end that all people may have better healthcare services. CNA's Web page contains news, links, industry facts, membership and job information.

Contact: e-mail directly from the site

 CAMPRN

Listproc@Listproc.wsu.edu

Discussion list for camp nurses, camp health professionals, and camp administrators to share information, resources, ideas, and experiences about camp health care. This list runs on the Listproc system. you will automatically be added to the list when you submit your request to join.

Subscribe CampRN Firstname Lastname

Canadian Association of Critical Care Nurses

www.caccn.ca

Website of the Canadian Association of Critical Care Nurses with information on membership, education, and research.

Contact: caccn@caccn.ca

 Canadian Intravenous Nurses Association

http://web.idirect.com/~csotcina/cina.html

Website of the Canadian Intravenous Nurses Association, which is an association that unites nurses initiating and maintaining IVs.

Contact: cinacscot@idirect.com

 Canadian Nurses Association

www.cna-nurses.ca/

Website of the Canadian Nurses Association. The site is available in both English and French.

Contact: cna@cna-nurses.ca

 CancerGuide: Steve Dunn's Cancer Information Page

www.cancerguide.org

A guide for cancer patients who want to understand and research the disease and their treatment options. The author is a cancer survivor himself.

Contact: Steve Dunn, dunn@cancerguide.org

CANCER-L

listserv@wvnvm.wvnet.edu

Discussion group on cancer and related issues. The list runs on the Listserv system. On subscribing, you will be asked to confirm your intention to join the list.

Subscribe CANCER-L Firstname Lastname

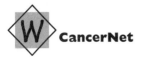 **CancerNet**

www.cancernet.nci.nih.gov

Maintained by the National Cancer Institute at the National Institutes of Health, this site contains extensive accurate, credible cancer information. All information located on CancerNet has been reviewed by oncology experts and is based on the results of current research.

Contact: webmaster@icic.nci.nih.gov

 CARENET

listserv@sco.georcoll.on.ca

International discussion group to explore issues of relevance to the development of Caring Theory and its application to nursing and nursing education. The list runs on the Listserv system. You will automatically added to list when you send your request to subscribe.

Subscribe CARENET Firstname Lastname

 CARENETL

listserv@admin.humberc.on.ca

Discussion group for nurse faculty. The list runs on the Listserv system. On subscribing, you will be asked to confirm your intention to join the list.

Subscribe CARENETL Firstname Lastname

Case Management Society of America

www.cmsa.org

The Case Management Society of America is an international, nonprofit organization dedicated to the support and development of the profession of case management through educational forums, networking opportunities, and legislative involvement. CMSA's success and strength is its structure as a member-driven society.

Contact: cmsa@cmsa.org

 CASEMGR

Casemgr-request@med-employ.com

Discussion list for case managers, as well as quality improvement and utilization review professionals. You will be added to the list automatically when you submit a request to join.

Subscribe (do not add your name)

 CATHAR-M

listserv@maelstrom.stjohns.edu

Electronically distributed newsmagazine for chronic fatigue syndrome. The list runs on the Listserv system. On subscribing, you will be asked to confirm your intention to join the list.

Subscribe CATHAR-M Firstname Lastname

 Catholic University of America School of Nursing

http://nursing.cua.edu

Comprehensive Website for the school of nursing, with courses, faculty, and resources.

Contact: cua-nursing@cua.edu

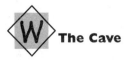 **The Cave**

www.uwm.edu/People/brodg/

Beth Rodgers is a faculty member at the University of WI-Milwaukee in the School of Nursing. The Cave was created in October 1997 as a major remodeling of her site, which had been active since mid-1995. The name is derived from Plato's famous allegory of the cave. Like humans living in a cave, often we are mistaken about what is real, believing that the shadows we see on the wall are, indeed, reality. For purposes here, the name is used to capture the ways in which the Internet provides us with a way to expand our boundaries beyond the walls of our own individual caves. This site was designed with the intent of providing easy access to starting points for nursing- and health-related sites, for computer and Internet information, and for some excellent philosophy and research-related sites.

Contact: Beth Rodgers, brodg@csd.uwm.edu

 Center for Applied Ethics and Professional Practice

www.edc.org/CAE/

This center designs, implements, and evaluates solutions to health and community problems, accomplishing change in ways that respect the often-conflicting values of our pluralistic society. A major current focus is on ensuring that scientific knowledge and new biomedical technologies, which carry with them the power both to do good and to do harm, are used wisely and effectively to improve the quality of life and the health of the public. Access the online journal *Innovations in End-of-Life Care* from this site.

Contact: Stacy A. Spiszcz, spiszcz@edc.org

 Center for Food Safety and Applied Nutrition

http://vm.cfsan.fda.gov/list.html

The Center for Food Safety and Applied Nutrition (CFSAN), regulates $240 billion worth of domestic food, $15 billion worth of imported foods, and $15 billion worth of cosmetics sold across state lines. This regulation takes place from the products' point of U.S. entry or processing to their point of sale. CFSAN is one of six centers within FDA. With a work force of about 800, the center promotes and protects the public health and economic interest by ensuring that food is safe, nutritious, and wholesome, and cosmetics are safe, and that food and cosmetics are honestly, accurately and informatively labeled. The CFSAN Website provides access to a variety of FDA publications and news alerts, covering such areas as food additives, biotechnology, food labeling, and food-borne illnesses.

Contact: Laurence Dusold, lrd@cfsan.fda.gov

 Center for Human Caring

www.uchsc.edu/ctrsinst/chc/index.htm

From the University of Colorado Health Sciences Center School of Nursing, this page is a collection of resources for those interested in the Center for Human Caring activities and Watson's theory of human caring.

Contact: Karen Holland, Karen.Holland@UCHSC.Edu

 Center for Narcolepsy Research

www.uic.edu/depts/cnr/

Information about narcolepsy from the Center for Narcolepsy Research, based at the College of Nursing, University of Illinois at Chicago. Includes links to other sleep resources.

Contact: narcolep@listserv.uic.edu

 Center for the Study of Autism (CSA)

www.autism.org

The Center for the Study of Autism is located in the Salem/Portland, Oregon area. The Center provides information about autism to parents and professionals, and conducts research on the efficacy of various therapeutic interventions. Much of their research is in collaboration with the Autism Research Institute. This site has links to detailed information on autism and related disorders, issues, and interventions. Basic information on autism is included in English, Chinese, Spanish, Italian, Japanese, and Korean.

Contact: samr7@netcom.com

Center for the Study of the History of Nursing

www.nursing.upenn.edu/history/

The Center for the Study of the History of Nursing was established in 1985 to encourage and facilitate historical scholarship on healthcare history and nursing in the United States. Now in its 15th year, the center continues to create and maintain a resource for such research, to improve the quality and scope of historical scholarship on nursing, and to disseminate new knowledge on nursing history through education, conferences, publications, and interdisciplinary collaboration.

Contact: nhistory@pobox.upenn.edu or e-mail directly from the site

 Centers for Disease Control and Prevention (CDC)

www.cdc.gov

CDC offers links to all of its centers, offices, and institutes; news alerts; and pointers to topics such as diseases, health risks, prevention guidelines and strategies, the Morbidity and Mortality Weekly Report, scientific data, health statistics, publications, and products.

Contact: inquiry@cdc.gov

 CenterWatch Clinical Trials Listing Service

www.centerwatch.com

A listing of more than 41,000 industry- and government-sponsored clinical trials as well as new drug therapies recently approved by the FDA. The site is designed to be a resource for patients interested in participating in clinical trials as well as for research professionals.

Contact: cntrwatch@aol.com

Centre for Evidence-Based Nursing

www.york.ac.uk/depts/hstd/centres/evidence/ev-intro.htm

From the University of York, The Centre for Evidence-Based Nursing is concerned with furthering evidence-based nursing through education, research, and development.

Contact: health-matters@york.ac.uk

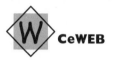 **CeWEB**

www.ce-web.com

Online continuing education (CE), brought to you by American Health Consultants, Inc. Topics covered include Quality/ Patient Management, Infection Control, and Outpatient and Home Health. There is a charge to take the tests and receive CE credit.

Contact: nurseinfo@ce-web.com

 CFS-L

listserv@maelstrom.stjohns.edu

Discussion group on chronic fatigue syndrome for patients and non-health professionals. The list runs on the Listserv system. Upon subscribing, you will be asked to confirm your intention to join the list.

Subscribe CFS-L Firstname Lastname

 CFS-MED

listserv@maelstrom.stjohns.edu

Discussion group on chronic fatigue syndrome for health professionals. The list runs on the Listserv system. You will be automatically added to the list when you submit a request to join.

Subscribe CFS-MED Firstname Lastname

CFS-NEWS

listserv@maelstrom.stjohns.edu

Electronic newsletter focusing on chronic fatigue syndrome. The list runs on the Listserv system. You will be automatically added to the list when you submit a request to join.

Subscribe CFS-NEWS Firstname Lastname

 Chronic Fatigue Syndrome/Myalgic Encephalomyelitis

www.cfs-news.org

An impressive collection of links to CFS resources on the Net; compiled by Roger Burns, publisher of the CFS-NEWS Electronic Newsletter. FAQs, informational articles, discussion groups, and magazines are among the resources covered here.

Contact: Roger Burns, cfs-news-request@maelstrom.stjohns.edu

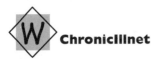 **ChronicIllnet**

www.chronicillnet.org

ChronicIllnet is a multimedia information source on the Internet dedicated to chronic illnesses including AIDS, cancer, Persian Gulf War syndrome, autoimmune diseases, chronic fatigue syndrome, heart disease, and neurological diseases. The information at this site is designed to appeal to a wide audience including researchers, physicians, and laypeople. New to the site are "Stories from the Frontline."

Contact: CIRFnet@aol.com

 CINAHL Information Systems

www.cinahl.com

The CINAHL Information Systems Website is a key access point to multidisciplinary professional literature. Products include the CINAHL database, a document delivery service, a literature search service, several print publications, the

Online Journal of Clinical Innovation, and CINAHL direct online service (membership fee).

Contact: support@cinahl.com

 Circumcision Information and Resource Pages

www.cirp.org

The Circumcision Information and Resource Pages are an Internet resource, providing information about all aspects of the genital surgery known as circumcision. CIRP is essentially divided into two parts: the circumcision reference library contains technical material, medical and historical articles, and statistics. The circumcision information pages contain a more readable collection of information, suitable for parents and educators. This site has links to information on the rights of the child, religious issues, and related issues.

Contact: Geoffrey T. Falk, cirp@cirp.org

 CLFORNSG

listserv@ulkyvm.louisville.edu

Discussion list for nurses interested in forensic nursing. The list runs on the Listserv system. You will be automatically added to the list when you submit a request to join.

Subscribe CLFORNSG Firstname Lastname

 Clinical Pharmacology 2000

www.cponline.gsm.com

Clinical Pharmacology 2000 provides information on all FDA-approved drugs and over-the-counter (OTC) pharmaceuticals. Herbal products and nutraceutical products are included when it appears that a reasonable amount of scientific data are available for review. Investigational drugs are included in the database when they have reached Phase III clinical investigation. All Clinical Pharmacology 2000 writers and editors are current or former clinical pharmacists who have been formally trained in drug information. No member of the editorial department has any direct relationship with any pharmaceutical manufacturer. This service is now free (registration required).

Contact: cponline@gsm.com

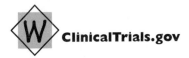 **ClinicalTrials.gov**

www.clinicaltrials.gov

The U.S. National Institutes of Health, through its National Library of Medicine, has developed ClinicalTrials.gov to provide patients, family members, and members of the public current information about clinical research studies.

Contact: e-mail directly from the site

 CNN Food and Health Main Page

www.cnn.com/HEALTH/

CNN presents features with full-text articles on the latest food and health news. Visitors can read the articles and hear sound bites from interviews. Topical chat forums are also available.

 CNS-L

listserv@listserv.utoronto.ca

Discussion group for clinical nurse specialists, affiliated with the CNS Interest Group of Ontario, Canada. The list runs on the Listserv system. Your request to join the list will be forwarded to the list owner for approval; once approved you will be added to the list without the necessity of sending a confirming response.

Subscribe CNS-L Firstname Lastname

 CNSA-L

listserv@listserv.utoronto.ca

CNSA-L is a discussion group for CNSA/AEIC, the national bilingual voice of nursing students in diploma and baccalaureate programs in Canada. The list runs on the Listserv system. On subscribing, you will be asked to confirm your intention to join the list.

Subscribe CNSA-L Firstname Lastname

 Cochrane Collaboration

www.cochrane.org.au

The Cochrane Collaboration is an international organization that aims to help people make well-informed decisions about health care by preparing, maintaining, and ensuring the accessibility of systematic reviews of the effects of healthcare interventions. The Collaboration is built on nine principles: collaboration, building on the enthusiasm of individuals, avoiding duplication, minimizing bias, keeping up to date, ensuring relevance, ensuring access, continually improving the quality of its work, and continuity. The Cochrane Library electronic disseminates the Collaboration's evidence-based practice databases electronically.

Contact: cochrane@med.monash.edu.au

 College of Nursing and Health Science at George Mason University

www.gmu.edu/departments/nursing/main.html

Visitors to this site can find information on programs in the college, as well as EDimensions, the college publication; information on the Center for Outcomes Research and Data Analysis; and the Center for Health Policy and Ethics.

Contact: Terry Ann Guingab, tguingab@gmu.edu

 COLON

listserv@listserv.acor.org

Discussion group on colon cancer and related issues. This list runs on the Listserv system. Upon subscribing, you will be asked to confirm your intention to join the list.

Subscribe COLON Firstname Lastname

Colorado Nurses' Association

www.sni.net/cna/

Website of the Colorado Nurses' Association, with legislative news, member information, a discussion forum, and listings of upcoming events.

Contact: Tim Brackett, RN, BSN, CNA@Nurses-CO.ORG

 Columbia University Gastroenterology Web

http://cpmcnet.columbia.edu/dept/gi/

A good starting point to link to other sites with gastroenterology and liver disease information on the Internet.

 Columbia University School of Nursing

http://cpmcnet.columbia.edu/dept/nursing/

Information on the School of Nursing at Columbia University in New York, with descriptions of programs, course listings, and faculty roster. The School now specializes in the education of nurses for advanced practice. The master's program, for nurses with a baccalaureate degree, prepares advanced practice nurses in eleven different clinical specializations. All of the master's programs allow graduates to be nationally certified in their area of specialization and to be registered with New York State as nurse practitioners. The doctoral program focuses on advanced clinical nursing practice and health services research.

Contact: sonadmit@columbia.edu

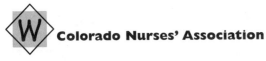 **Community of Science Web Server**

www.cos.com

Community of Science, Inc. (COS) is a network of Websites for scholars, scientists, and R&D professionals. The site contains information about scientific expertise, funded scientific research, and funding opportunities for research. The COS philosophy is to provide working researchers with valuable information tools to help them complete work under way and secure funds for the next project. COS is a consortium of research institutions and one of the largest repositories of searchable scientific information available on the Internet.

Computer Related Repetitive Strain Injury

www.engr.unl.edu/ee/eeshop/rsi.html

Tips for avoiding repetitive strain injury (RSI) are found at this site, which also offers diagrams of proper typing position, descriptions of the first warning signs of injury, and resource links. The author of the page is Paul Marxhausen, an engineering electronics technician who has suffered from RSI since March 1994.

Contact: Paul Marxhausen, pmarxhausen@unl.edu

Cool Nursing Site of the Week

www.microtec.net/fnord/nurselink.html

New sites appear on the Internet daily. Visit the cool nursing site of the week to find out what is new, and cool, on the Web. Although the site appears to be updated less than weekly, it is still a good resource for nursing links.

Contact: Thomas Moll, fnord@microtec.net

Cornucopia of Disability Information (CODI)

http://codi.buffalo.edu/

CODI serves as a community resource for consumers and professionals by providing disability information in a wide variety of areas. The information addresses university (State University of New York at Buffalo), local (Buffalo and western New York), state, national, and international audiences. Submissions are welcome from these communities. Areas include education, directories and databases, statistics, government documents, computer access, legal, publications, WWW, bibliographic references, aging, politics, universal design, and announcements.

Contact: Jennifer Weir, jweir@acsu.buffalo.edu

Country Joe McDonald's Tribute to Florence Nightingale

www.dnai.com/~borneo/nightingale/

You have to see this site to believe it. The singer Country Joe McDonald has become a student of the life of Florence Nightingale. This site includes a history of Miss Nightingale, a picture of Country Joe's nurse doll collection, and a memorial to women who died in the Vietnam War. The entire site is beautifully done, with many pictures and a recording of Miss Nightingale, made in 1890 (the same recording that is available at InterNurse).

Contact: Country Joe McDonald, joe@countryjoe.com

C-PALSY

listserv@maelstrom.stjohns.edu

Discussion group about cerebral palsy and related issues. This list runs on the Listserv system. On subscribing, you will be asked to confirm your intention to join the list.

Subscribe C-PALSY Firstname Lastname

Critical Care Nurse Snapshots

www.nursing.umaryland.edu/students/~jkohl/scenario/opening.htm

Critical Care Nurse Snapshots are designed to be interactive case scenarios for nurses involved in making informed decisions at the bedside. Each case study involves the student in the critical thinking process as it relates to the assessment, diagnosis, management, and follow-up of a clinically based problem.

Contact: James E. Kohl, jkohl@umabnet.ab.umd.edu

CTNURS-L

listserv@uconnvm.uconn.edu

Discussion list for the nurses of Connecticut. This list runs on the Listserv system. On subscribing, you will be asked to confirm your intention to join the list.

Subscribe CTNURS-L Firstname Lastname

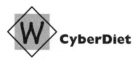 **CyberDiet**

www.cyberdiet.com

CyberDiet, "the best place to go to answer all your questions about adopting a healthy lifestyle," is the work of cofounders Timi Gustafson, RD, and Cynthia Fink. The site offers highly interactive modules that allow its users to customize a program to achieve their specific goals, and it provides vast nutritional information at the click of a mouse. CyberDiet offers its visitors a means of achieving their specific goals through extensive use of online interactive modules as well as detailed nutritional information and motivation.

Contact: eatright@cyberdiet.com

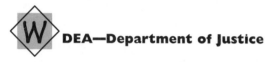 **DEA—Department of Justice**

www.usdoj.gov/dea/

Website for the Drug Enforcement Agency (DEA) of the Department of Justice. It includes information on the mission of the DEA, programs, education, drugs of concern, and fugitives. Information regarding distribution of controlled substances for medicinal purposes can be found under "Diversion Control" in the programs section.

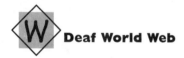 **Deaf World Web**

www.deafworldweb.org

Deaf and hearing people alike can click into the world of the deaf at this expanding site. The site includes news, art, discussion and chat areas, information for children, and an interactive American Sign Language (ASL) dictionary. A Web pioneer, this site has been online since February 1995.

Contact: dww@dww.org

Dee's Pain Management Page

www.web-shack.com/dee/

Dee Burrows is a nurse, lecturer, and researcher at Buckinghamshire College of Nursing and Midwifery. Her Website includes her own experience with and research on pain management, information on the Pain Interest Group of South Buckinghamshire, and other nursing and pain management links.

Contact: Dee Burrows, dee@ptop.demon.co.uk

 Diabetes Mall on the Net

www.diabetesnet.com

The Diabetes Mall provides a weekly online diabetes newspaper, Diabetes This Week, plus research reports, articles analyzing current diabetes issues, interactive tools for better blood sugar control, contests, and information on the latest drugs, medications, devices, products, diets, blood sugar management tools, and future developments in diabetes care. The online store offers diabetes books, software, scales, and other products to educate, entertain, and inform.

Contact: contact@diabetesnet.com

 différance: Peter Murray's Website

www.lemmus.demon.co.uk/diff01.htm

This Website has links to nursing informatics topics related to nursing and healthcare informatics, journals, people, and sites. Also includes, among others, links to the Betty Neuman page with information about the theorist and the Neuman Systems Model.

Contact: peter@nursing-informatics.net

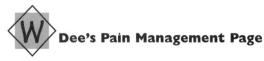 **Digital Anatomist Project**

http://sig.biostr.washington.edu/projects/da/

The University of Washington's virtual anatomy lab, with hundreds of images.

Contact: digital_anatomist@biostr.washington.edu

disABILITY Information and Resources

www.eskimo.com/~jlubin/disabled.html

A comprehensive list of disability-related links. The pages provided are intended as a resource to provide useful information, are not graphics intensive, and therefore are quick to load. The site was created and is maintained solely by Jim Lubin, who is a C2 quadriplegic, completely paralyzed from the neck down and dependent on a ventilator to breathe. He uses a keyboard/mouse emulator with a sip and puff switch to type Morse codes.

Contact: Jim Lubin, jlubin@eskimo.com

 Disability Link Barn

www.accessunlimited.com/links.html

A site of over 100 links for people with disabilities of all types. The site is well organized and comprehensive. It is maintained by Access Unlimited, a manufacturer and distributor of adaptive transportation and mobility equipment for people with disabilities.

Contact: info@accessunlimited.com

 Diseases, Disorders and Related Topics

www.mic.ki.se/Diseases/index.html

An exhaustive collection of resources for laypeople, healthcare professionals, and scientists involved in the study or treatment of diseases, disorders, or any number of related medical issues. Whether your specialty is bacterial, behavioral, viral, or parasitic, in the realm of animal diseases, anesthesia, surgery, or dentistry, the Karolinska Institute's Diseases, Disorders and Related Topics is sure to cover it. Of special interest is a humanities section exploring ethics in medicine.

Contact: info@kib.ki.se

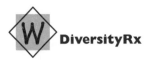 **DiversityRx**

www.diversityrx.org

DiversityRx promotes language and cultural competence to improve the quality of health care for minority, immigrant, and ethnically diverse communities. This site has many resources in support of that mission.

Contact: rcchc@aol.com

 drkoop.com

www.drkoop.com

Consumer-oriented Website led by C. Everett Koop, former U.S. Surgeon General. As one of the most visited health sites on the Web, it represents one of the many sources of information for patients.

Contact: feedback@drkoop.com

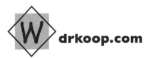 **Duke University School of Nursing**

http://son3.mc.duke.edu/

This Website has program, faculty, educational resources, and contact information at the Duke University School of Nursing.

Contact: Jacqueline Nelson, nelson031@mc.duke.edu

 East Tennessee State University College of Nursing

www.etsu.edu/etsucon/

This Website has program information, news, and nursing-related links.

Contact: riddles@etsu.edu

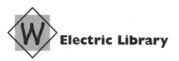 **Electric Library**

www.elibrary.com

The Electric Library is a searchable database. You can pose a question in plain English and launch a comprehensive, simultaneous search through hundreds of full-text newspapers, magazines, newswires, books, maps, photographs, and major works of literature and art. To use this search engine, you must subscribe to the service, and there is a fee, although 30-day trial subscriptions are available.

Contact: elibrary@infonautics.com

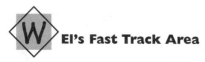 **El's Fast Track Area**

www.geocities.com/HotSprings/1003/

Eleanor Elston is a registered nurse who has worked in emergency, critical care, and community health nursing in British Columbia. Her Website includes a variety of nursing links, personal information, and some humorous sites.

Contact: eelston@iname.com

 Emergency Medicine and Primary Care Website

www.embbs.com

Educational resources for emergency and primary care providers. The site includes radiologic images, CT scan and medical photograph libraries, clinical cases—see if you can make the diagnosis—and megacode simulators.

Contact: Ash Nashed, MD, ashrafn@aol.com

 Emergency Nurses Association (ENA)

www.ena.org

The ENA Website highlights information about the association, the ENA foundation, the Board of Certification for Emergency Nursing, and EN CARE (Cancel Alcohol Related Emergencies).

Contact: enainfo@ena.org

Emergency Nursing World

http://enw.org

Lots of information, resources, and links for nurses in emergency practice.

Contact: Tom Trimble, RN, tom@enw.org

 EM-NSG-L

listserv@itssrv1.ucsf.edu

Discussion list for emergency nurses. The list runs on the Listserv system. On subscribing, you will be asked to confirm your intention of joining the list.

Subscribe EM-NSG-L Firstname Lastname

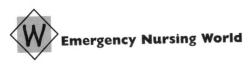 **Emory University's MedWeb: Biomedical Internet Resources**

www.medweb.emory.edu/medweb/

Emory University's MedWeb is a list of more than 8,000 links to health information Web pages, with an extensive catalog of specialties. The nursing page has links to schools of nursing and career directories, Websites, documents, and electronic newsletters and journals.

Contact: medweb@emory.edu

 Epilepsy Foundation

www.efa.org

Website for the Epilepsy Foundation. The site includes information for patients, family members, and health professionals in the areas of research, advocacy, education, and service. There is information on the Gene Discovery Project and teen and children's areas.

Contact: webmaster@efa.org

EPILEPSY-L

listserv@home.ease.lsoft.com

Discussion group about epilepsy and seizure disorders. The list runs on the List-serv system. On receipt of your request to subscribe, you will be asked to confirm your intention to join the list.

Subscribe EPILEPSY-L Firstname Lastname

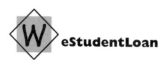 **eStudentLoan**

www.estudentloan.com

"eStudentLoan is a marketplace where students and parents can match their specific needs with what various lenders can provide. eStudentLoan provides a unique service on the Web—we are the only site that is a universal resource for information about student loans—whether GOVT Loans, Alternative loans, loans in a student's name, or loans in a parent's name. eStudentLoan is the only Web-based organization keeping track of the inner workings of the alternative student loan world and passing that valuable information to students and parents in search of financial aid."

Contact: customerservice@estudentloan.com

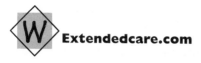 **Extendedcare.com**

www.extendedcare.com

Extendedcare.com offers Internet-based solutions and resources that connect hospitals, consumers and extended care providers (such as nursing, assisted living and other senior living facilities, and home healthcare agencies) to each other. Founded by healthcare professionals, extendedcare.com has products and services intended to improve the discharge planning process for hospitals, enhance the admissions process for extended care providers, and assist consumers in finding extended care providers and information on senior health issues.

Contact: ecininc@ecininc.com

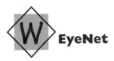 **EyeNet**

www.eyenet.org

An education and reference site maintained by the American Academy of Ophthalmology, an international member association of more than 21,000 specialists.

Contact: comm@aao.org

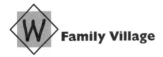 **Family Village**

www.familyvillage.wisc.edu

The Family Village is a global community that integrates information, resources, and communication opportunities on the Internet for persons with cognitive and other disabilities, their families, and those who provide them services and supports. The Family Village Website has a well-rounded offering of information for disabled persons including medical, educational, spiritual, and recreational resources.

Contact: familyvillage@waisman.wisc.edu

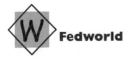 **Fedworld**

http://fedworld.gov

A U.S. government–maintained database of documents and resources on a wide variety of topics including health, medicine, and nursing.

 Fibromyalgia Resources

www.hsc.missouri.edu/~fibro

The Missouri Arthritis Rehabilitation Research and Training Center has created this Website as an educational resource for patients and physicians. This site has fibromyalgia FAQs for patients and healthcare providers, other education resources, and information about the organization.

Contact: marrtc@health.missouri.edu

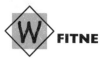 **FITNE**

www.fitne.net

FITNE promotes the use of technology in healthcare education by developing and distributing multimedia hardware systems and software. The Website has information on the conferences, products, seminars, and more.

Contact: fitne@ev.net

 Florida Atlantic University College of Nursing

www.fau.edu/divdept/nursing/

This site includes a description of programs, faculty listing with research interests, and back issues of "Nightingale Songs," a publication that allows nurses to share esthetic expressions about their nursing experiences.

Contact: boykina@fau.edu

 Florida International University School of Nursing

www.fiu.edu/orgs/nursing/

Informational site with course descriptions, faculty listing, and programs. The site also includes information on a number of nursing theories and a bibliography of readings on Orem.

Contact: Douglas Coffin, PhD, ARNP, coffin@fiu.edu

 Florida State University School of Nursing

www.fsu.edu/~nursing/Nursing.html

This site has information on the degree programs, course requirements, faculty, and a description and history of the school of nursing.

Contact: smt2485@mailer.fsu.edu

Fort Hays State University School of Nursing

www.fhsu.edu/nursing/

This site includes information on courses, programs, and faculty, as well as distance education.

Contact: Elaine Diehl, ediehl@fhsu.edu

 Frances Payne Bolton School of Nursing

http://fpb.cwru.edu

Visitors here can learn about the Frances Payne Bolton School of Nursing at Case Western Reserve University. The site includes information from the general bulletin, faculty listing, degree programs, and curriculum information.

Contact: webmaster@fpb.cwru.edu

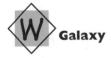 **Galaxy**

www.einet.net/galaxy.html

Galaxy is a guide to worldwide services and information. The site provides links to many topics of interest, including business, community, engineering, government, humanities, law, leisure, medicine, reference, science, and the social sciences. Although many of the links from the nursing section have been explored and included elsewhere in this directory, this is a good site to connect to many other areas of information.

Contact: webmaster@galaxy.com

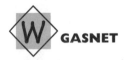 **GASNET**

www.gasnet.org

GASNET is a global anesthesiology server network for reference and education that includes abstracts from several journals; a video library, a discussion group, and commercial software demonstrations; an e-mail directory; and links to many other anesthesiology resources on the Internet.

Contact: webmaster@www.gasnet.org

GENERAL COMMUNITY HEALTH ISSUES

listserv@zeus.med.uottawa.ca

Discussion group for community health professionals. The list runs on the Listserv system. On subscribing, you will be asked to confirm your intention of joining the list.

Contact: Subscribe general_community_health_issues Firstname Lastname

 General Practice On-Line

www.priory.com

The site of the journal *General Practice On-Line*, a peer-reviewed electronic journal with articles for primary care providers. There are also links to other electronic journals published by Priory Lodge Education, including *Chest Medicine On-Line, Psychiatry On-Line, Family Medicine On-Line,* and *History of Medicine On-Line,* among others.

 GERINET

listserv@listserv.acsu.buffalo.edu

Discussion group for geriatric care, gerontology, and related issues. The list runs on the Listserv system. On subscribing, you will be asked to confirm your intention to join the list.

Subscribe GERINET Firstname Lastname

 GERO-NURSE

GERO-NURSE-REQUEST@list.uiowa.edu

Listserv for the Research Development and Dissemination Core at the University of Iowa Gerontological Nursing Intervention Research Center. Requests to join are forwarded to the list owner; once approved, you will be automatically added to the list.

Subscribe

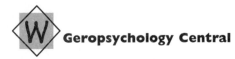 **Geropsychology Central**

www.premier.net/~gero/geropsyc.html

Geropsychology Central provides links to information and services for older adults and geropsychology professionals, covering neurological, psychological, and sociological aspects of aging.

Contact: gero@premier.net

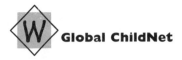 **Global ChildNet**

http://edie.cprost.sfu.ca/gcnet/index.html

Global ChildNet, with its headquarters in Vancouver, BC, was officially introduced at the Child Health 2000 World Congress. It is an organization that uses the Internet to offer a range of easily accessible, child health–related online services. These services include databases and other information on issues related to the well-being of the world's children. As a division of the Global Child Health Society, a nonprofit organization, Global ChildNet also publishes an online version of the *Global Child Health News and Review*, as well as supplying information on the Child Health 2000 World Congress and Exposition. By using state-of-the-art technology, Global ChildNet complements the newspaper and the congress to provide worldwide networking for health professionals, child health workers, scientists, nongovernmental organizations, health planners, and child advocates.

Contact: gcnet@unixg.ubc.ca

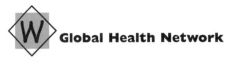 **Global Health Network**

www.pitt.edu/HOME/GHNet/GHNet.html

The mission of the Global Health Network (GHN) is to develop a worldwide network of people engaged in public health and disease prevention. Information at the site is available in Japanese, Spanish, Portuguese, German, Chinese, Turkish, and Taiwanese, as well as English.

Contact: Amy Brenen brenena@ghnet.org

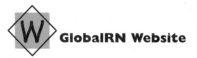 **GlobalRN Website**

http://nurseweb.ucsf.edu/www/globalrn.htm

GLOBALRN is a worldwide Internet e-mail discussion list on culture and healthcare issues. This Website is maintained by the list owner (supervisor) of GLOBALRN to highlight World Wide Web resources of interest in these subject areas. Instructions for joining the list are available at this site.

Contact: Chuck Pitkofsy, chuckp@itsa.ucsf.edu

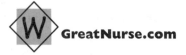 **GreatNurse.com**

www.greatnurse.com

GreatNurse.com offers free job classifieds to the nursing community. Positions are categorized by location (state, country, or region). You can enter a key word into the word search to further enhance your search.

Contact: feedback@greatnurse.com

 Greyhound-L

listserv@apple.ease.lsoft.com

Exclusively dedicated to Greyhounds, both retired racers and others. The list runs on the Listserv system. On subscribing, you will be asked to confirm your intention to join the list.

Subscribe Greyhound-L Firstname Lastname

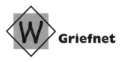 **Griefnet**

www.rivendell.org/

GriefNet is an Internet community of persons dealing with grief, death, and major loss. It has 37 e-mail support groups. Its integrated approach to online grief support provides help to people working through loss and grief issues. A companion site, KIDSAID, provides a safe environment for kids and their parents to find information and ask questions. GriefNet is supervised by Cendra (ken'dra) Lynn, PhD, a clinical grief psychologist, death educator, and traumatologist.

Contact: webmaster@griefnet.org

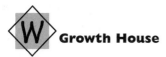 **Growth House**

www.growthhouse.org

This Website is an international gateway to resources for life-threatening illness and end-of-life care. Its primary mission is to improve the quality of compassionate care for people who are dying through public education and global professional collaboration.

Contact: info@growthhouse.org

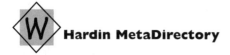 **Hardin MetaDirectory**

www.lib.uiowa.edu/hardin/md/

"We list the best sites that list the sites." The original and perhaps the most complete index on the Web. Brought to you courtesy of the Hardin Library for the Health Sciences at the University of Iowa.

Contact: hardin-webmaster@uiowa.edu

 HCARENURS

Majordomo@po.cwru.edu

Discussion group for home care nurses. The list runs on the Majordomo system. On subscribing, you will be asked to confirm your intention of joining the list.

Subscribe HCARENURS Firstname Lastname

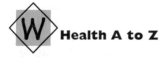 **Health A to Z**

www.healthatoz.com

This family health site includes extensive health information and news. It is a consumer-oriented site with a slick design and lots of information and links.

Contact: info@healthatoz.com

Health Information Research Unit

http://hiru.mcmaster.ca/

The Health Information Research Unit at McMaster University conducts research in the field of health information science and is dedicated to the generation of new knowledge about the nature of health and clinical information problems, the development of new information resources to support evidence-based health care, and the evaluation of various innovations in overcoming healthcare information problems.

Contact: amurray@fhs.mcmaster.ca

 Health On the Net Foundation

www.hon.ch/

An international initiative, Health On the Net Foundation is a not-for-profit organization, headquartered in Geneva, Switzerland. The foundation is dedicated to realizing the benefits of the Internet and related technologies in the fields of medicine and health care. With private and public sector support, the foundation actively promotes effective Internet use and demonstrates best-in-class implementation and application. Visitors to this site can use MedHunt, a multilingual search engine of thousands of health Websites.

Contact: webmaster@hon.ch

 Health Promotion Online (HPO)

www.hc-sc.gc.ca/hppb/hpo/

From Health Canada, HPO supports the development and coordination of health promotion and disease prevention programs. The site addresses a wide range of issues including workplace safety, physical activity, HIV/AIDS, aging, hepatitis C, cancer, tobacco, alcohol and other drugs, nutrition, and more.

Contact: hpo@hc-sc.gc.ca

Health Resources on IHP Net

www.ihpnet.org/4health.html

This site is designed to save time with presurfed, direct routes to health information you can use now. The locations have been designed to cut through the layers to within only a click or two of truly useful data.

Contact: ulysses@ihpnet.org

 Healthcare Financing Administration (HCFA)

www.hcfa.gov

Visitors to the Medicare and Medicaid site will find such resources as Healthcare Review, HCFA Health Watch, and research and demonstration initiatives.

Contact: webmaster@hcfa.gov

 Healthcare Information Technology Yellow Pages

www.health-infosys-dir.com

The Healthcare Information Technology Yellow Pages provides one-stop shopping for hospitals, clinics, health maintenance organizations (HMOs), preferred provider organizations (PPOs), and other healthcare providers. Research leading IT companies and consultants. The "White Pages" section includes comprehensive reports.

Contact: info@olcsoft.com

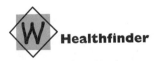 **Healthfinder**

www.healthfinder.gov

Healthfinder is a gateway consumer health and human services information Website from the U.S. Department of Health and Human Services. Healthfinder can lead you to selected online publications, clearinghouses, databases, Websites, and support and self-help groups, as well as the government agencies and not-for-profit organizations that produce reliable information for the public.

Contact: healthfinder@health.org

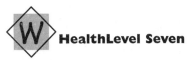 **HealthLevel Seven**

http://www.hl7.org/

This is the home page for HealthLevel Seven (HL7), one of several ANSI-accredited Standards Developing Organizations (SDOs) operating in the healthcare arena. There is comprehensive information on events, membership, resources, and committees available at the site.

Contact: hq@hl7.org

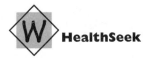 **HealthSeek**

www.healthseek.com

HealthSeek is a commercial online healthcare information service, providing healthcare professionals, consumers, and companies with a central site for obtaining news, information, and resources.

Contact: webmaster@healthseek.com

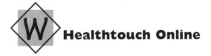 **Healthtouch Online**

www.healthtouch.com

Healthtouch Online brings together information from various health organizations. Visitors to this page may conduct searches to find drug information or listings (not necessarily complete) of local pharmacies. The Health Resource Directory lists and links health organizations and health government agencies.

Contact: e-mail directly from the site

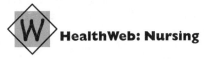 **HealthWeb: Nursing**

www.lib.umich.edu/hw/nursing.html

This page is a collaborative effort of the Taubman Medical Library, the School of Nursing at the University of Michigan, and the HealthWeb project. From this page, nurses can connect to career information, clinical nursing resources, interactive forums, academic programs, professional associations, electronic journals, and the HealthWeb.

Contact: nursingpage@umich.edu

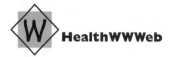

HealthWWWeb

www.healthwwweb.com

HealthWWWeb: Choices for Health is a site that combines integrative medicine, natural health, and alternative therapies. The site includes information on nutrition and healing therapies and links to other health-oriented sites on the Web.

Contact: webmaster@HealthWWWeb.com

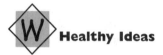

Healthy Ideas

www.healthyideas.com

Healthy Ideas is brought to you by *Prevention Magazine,* the popular health magazine. It provides extensive consumer-oriented health and home strategies and tips.

Healthy People 2010

http://web.health.gov/healthypeople/

Healthy People is a national health promotion and disease prevention initiative that brings together national, state, and local government agencies; nonprofit, voluntary, and professional organizations; businesses; communities; and individuals to improve the health of all Americans, eliminate disparities in health, and improve years and quality of healthy life. The site includes information on the prevention agenda, what you can do, and measuring progress.

Contact: HPWebsite@osophs.dhhs.gov

HEM-ONC

listserv@listserv.acor.org

Discussion group for hematologic oncology. It is professionally oriented. The list runs on the Listserv system. On subscribing, you will be asked to confirm your intention to join the list.

Subscribe HEM-ONC Firstname Lastname

 Hepnet: The Hepatitis Information Network

www.hepnet.com

This site focuses on the needs of the medical community, providing updates on patient care issues, serology, new clinical papers, quizzes, and news releases, as well as patient information and links to many other excellent hepatitis-related sites.

Contact: webmaster@hepnet.com

 HighWire Press

http://highwire.stanford.edu

HighWire Press, the Internet imprint of the Stanford University Libraries, is one of the two largest archives of free full-text science on earth, currently assisting in the online publication of 171,310 free full-text articles and 653,301 total articles.

Contact: contact@highwire.stanford.edu

 HIMSS—Healthcare Information and Management Systems Society

www.himss.org

"HIMSS is a not-for-profit organization representing information and management systems professionals in healthcare, serving our members, our customers, and our industry by providing leadership, education, and networking." The Website includes news, an online job search for healthcare information professionals, the Journal of Healthcare Information Management online, and a discussion forum.

Contact: himss@himss.org

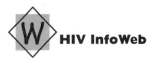 **HIV InfoWeb**

http://www.aegis.com/hivinfoweb/

The HIV InfoWeb is a nonprofit organization affiliated with the Justice Resource Institute. "We believe people should be able to take control of their medical treatment, to whatever degree they desire; we believe no one needs to become a full-time AIDS activist in order to take that control; we believe in the principle of democracy of information; everyone should be able to post their version of the truth, and let others decide for themselves what part of that truth they are going to adopt; we believe in the vision of a virtual community. 'Virtual' community means, a 'substantial, effective' community. You can join this community simply by using the resources of the Internet. And we will all benefit by each other's presence there."

 HODGKINS

listserv@solar.org

Discussion group on Hodgkin's disease and related lymphomas. The list runs on the Listserv system. On subscribing, you will be asked to confirm your intention to join the list.

Subscribe HODGKINS (do not follow by typing your name)

 Home Healthcare Nurses Association

www.nahc.org/HHNA/

Website of the Home Healthcare Nurses Association, a national nursing organization of individual members who are involved in home healthcare practice, education, administration, and research. News, events, and membership information are available at the site.

Contact: hhna_info@nahc.org

HOMEHLTH

listserv@usa.net

Discussion group on home health care and related issues. The list runs on the Listserv system. On subscribing, you will be asked to confirm your intention to join the list.

Subscribe HOMEHLTH Firstname Lastname

 Home Page of Susan K. Newbold

http://nursing.umaryland.edu/~snewbol/

Susan K. Newbold's Website has information on CARING (Capital Area Round-table on Informatics in NursinG), links to nursing informatics and health informatics conferences, and lists of nursing informatics groups around the world. A visitor here can also link to organizational information on the Pi Chapter of Sigma Theta Tau International Nursing Honor Society.

Contact: Susan Newbold, snewbold@umaryland.edu

 Hospice Foundation of America

www.hospicefoundation.org

On this page you can learn about hospice care, how to select a hospice, and how to locate a hospice near you. You can learn of the Hospice Foundation's programs, read excerpts from their publications, order books and videos, and sign up for the annual bereavement teleconference.

Contact: hfa@hospicefoundation.org

 Hospice Hands

http://hospice-cares.com

An online hospice community, sponsored by Hospice of North Central Florida. Lots of resources about hospice and more than 650 links to other hospice sites.

Contact: healing@hospice-cares.com

Hospice and Palliative Nurses Association

www.hpna.org

Website of the Hospice and Palliative Nurses Association. Membership, certification information, lists of courses and events, and links to additional resources are featured.

Contact: hnafan@pipeline.com

 HospitalWeb

http://neuro-www.mgh.harvard.edu/hospitalweb.shtml

HospitalWeb is a growing list of hospitals on the Web. Providing a simple and globally accessible way for patients, medical researchers, and physicians to get information on any hospital in the world is the goal. This list is of "main" Web servers (only Web servers at hospitals) as opposed to departments within hospitals. The site is maintained by the Department of Neurology at Massachusetts General Hospital.

Contact: prady@helix.mgh.harvard.edu

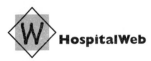 **Human Anatomy Online**

www.innerbody.com

A colorful, interactive human anatomy site. You can explore body systems that include full descriptions and other related illustrations.

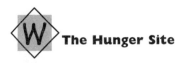 **The Hunger Site**

www.hungersite.com

The Hunger Site is an innovative new tool to help feed the hungry through the United Nations World Food Programme (WFP). Visitors to the site are invited to clicking on a button to donate food, which is paid for by corporate sponsors. The money received helps WFP provide desperately needed food assistance to hungry people in 80 countries. Between June 1999 and January 2000, more than 9 million pounds of food, equivalent to nearly 75 million cups, have gone to feed the hungry as a result of the nearly 34 million visitors who have visited The Hunger Site and clicked to help the hungry.

Contact: comments@thehungersite.com

 Idaho State University Department of Nursing

www.isu.edu/departments/nursing/

Highlights of this Website include information on the nursing program, online catalog, faculty, as well as a student thesis database.

Contact: taylrand@isu.edu

 IMMUNE

immune-request@lists.best.com

Support and information about multiple chemical sensitivities, chronic fatigue syndrome, fibromyalgia, lupus, multiple sclerosis, porphyria, allergies, asthma, and other immune-related ailments. The list runs on the Bestserv system. On subscribing, you will be asked to confirm your intention of joining the list.

Subscribe (do not type your name)

 Immunization Action Coalition

www.immunize.org

Immunization Action Coalition, a 501(c)3 nonprofit organization, works to boost immunization rates in the United States. The Coalition promotes physician, community, and family awareness of and responsibility for appropriate immunization of all people of all ages against all vaccine-preventable diseases. The coalition's Website provides electronic versions of its newsletters, Needle Tips and Hepatitis B Coalition News, as well as quizzes, news, and extensive health links.

Contact: admin@immunize.org

Indiana Prevention Resource Center

www.drugs.indiana.edu

The center offers information about alcohol, tobacco, and drug abuse, including a dictionary of slang terms, abbreviations, and acronyms compiled by the Indiana Prevention Resource Center and the National Drugs and Crime Clearinghouse files. Major headings include Prevention, Drug Information, Statistics, Publications, and Resources.

Contact: drugprc@indiana.edu

 Indiana University School of Nursing-Bloomington

www.indiana.edu/~iubnurse

The Indiana University School of Nursing Website has information on its academic programs, faculty, the Association of Nursing Students, and a bulletin board for students. There are also links to nursing-related Websites and sites of general interest.

Contact: iubnurse@indiana.edu

 Indiana University School of Nursing-Indianapolis

www.iupui.edu/~nursing/

Indiana University School of Nursing (IUSON) is an academic community that is internationally known for the excellence and diversity of its programs. One of the top-ranked and largest schools of nursing in the United States, IUSON awards the full range of academic degrees, from the associate to doctoral level, and offers courses on eight campuses throughout the state of Indiana as well as via distance learning.

Contact: Louise Watkins, lwatkin@iupui.edu

INDIE: The Integrated Network of Disability Information and Education

http://indie.ca

INDIE facilitates the sharing of disability-related information to foster a collaborative approach to addressing disability issues among Canadians with disabilities and their organizations. This site is bilingual (English/French).

Contact: webmaster@indie.ca

 In-Hospital Defibrillation

www.defib.net

Should nurses perform defibrillation? Read some views and issues at this site to make up your mind.

Contact: John Stewart, RN, MA, jastewart@defib.net

 International Association for the Study of Pain (IASP)

www.halcyon.com/iasp/

The purposes of this Website are to introduce healthcare professionals and scientists to IASP, to provide services and resources to IASP members, to provide a vehicle for the educational outreach of IASP, to call attention to the importance of pain as a field for multidisciplinary scientific inquiry, and to make pain prevention and relief a priority for healthcare delivery.

Contact: iasp@locke.hs.washington.edu

 International Cancer Alliance for Research and Education (ICARE)

www.icare.org

The International Cancer Alliance for Research and Education (ICARE) is a non-profit organization that provides high-quality, focused, user-friendly, cancer information to each patient as well as their physician on an on-going, person-to-person basis. ICARE has developed several unique patient-centered programs through an extensive process of collection, evaluation, and dissemination of information, bringing the cancer patient in contact with top physicians and scientists from around the world. This organization is operated by a network of people scientists, clinicians, caring staff and lay volunteers, many of whom are patients themselves.

Contact: info@icare.org

 International Committee of the Red Cross

www.icrc.org

A look at the work of the International Committee of the Red Cross, based in Geneva, Switzerland. The ICRC server features extensive information on Red Cross operations worldwide; the mission, philosophy, and strategic operations of the ICRC; issues and topics of concern to the organization; and a full explanation of International Humanitarian Law, including the full texts of the Geneva Conventions. English, French, and Spanish language editions of the site are available.

Contact: webmaster.gva@icrc.org

 International Federation of MS Societies (IFMSS)

www.ifmss.org.uk

IFMSS is a nongovernmental, nonprofit voluntary health agency and umbrella organization for the 34 established national MS member societies throughout the world. One of the major IFMSS objectives is to serve as a clearinghouse for educational and scientific information about MS. The World of Multiple Sclerosis (WoMS) is an international cooperative effort using experts in all areas of MS to offer current and useful information to all members of the MS community (health professionals, researchers, persons with MS, families, and caregivers), as well as the general public. The annotated directory has links to news and updates, research, user and support groups, publications, and other useful information.

Contact: webmaster, psherida@mail.usyd.edu.au

International Food Information Council

http://ificinfo.health.org

The purpose of the International Food Information Council (IFIC) Foundation is to bridge the gap between science and communications by collecting and disseminating scientific information on food safety, nutrition, and health and by working with an extensive roster of scientific experts to help translate research into understandable and useful information for opinion leaders and, ultimately, consumers. These groups find the IFIC reservoir of science and health data a valuable and easily accessed resource. Information available includes scientific research, informational materials, graphics, and other information on a broad range of food issues. Some highlights include tips for educators and consumers, a section containing information for reporters, and answers to frequently asked food-related questions.

Contact: foodinfo@ific.health.org

 International Nurses Society on Addictions

www.nnsa.org or www.intnsa.org

The International Nurses Society on Addictions (IntNSA) is a professional specialty organization founded in 1975 (as the National Nurses Society on Addictions) for nurses committed to the prevention, intervention, treatment, and management of addictive disorders. The Website offers news, position statements, conference schedules, links, and certification information.

Contact: webmaster@intnsa.org

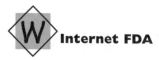 **Internet FDA**

www.fda.gov

Assessing risks—and, for drugs and medical devices, weighing risks against benefits—is at the core of the FDA's public health protection duties. By ensuring that products and producers meet certain standards, the FDA protects consumers and enables us to know what we are buying. Main headings on the site include foods, human drugs, biologics, animal drugs, cosmetics, medical devices/radiological health, freedom of information, field operations, children and tobacco, toxicology research, and med watch.

Contact: webmail@oc.fda.gov

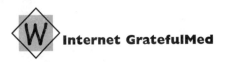 **Internet GratefulMed**

http://igm.nlm.nih.gov

Internet GratefulMed offers assisted searching in MEDLINE and other online databases of the U.S. National Library of Medicine (NLM). It was developed through the User Access Services project of NLM's System Reinvention initiative. Internet GratefulMed can map user terms through NLM's Unified Medical Language System (UMLS). The Metathesaurus helps users create, submit, and refine a search in MEDLINE. Searching MEDLINE using Internet GratefulMed is free.

Contact: Internet GratefulMed Development Team, access@nlm.nih.gov

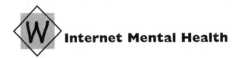 **Internet Mental Health**

www.mentalhealth.com

Internet Mental Health is a free encyclopedia of mental health information. It was developed by a Canadian psychiatrist, Phillip W. Long, and programmed by his colleague Brian Chow. Internet Mental Health is designed to promote improved understanding, diagnosis, and treatment of mental illness throughout the world.

Contact: editor@mentalhealth.com

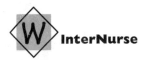 **InterNurse**

www.internurse.com

This site is designed to bring a sense of a nursing magazine to the Internet. There are many wonderful nurse-related sites and groups on the Internet; Inter-Nurse provides coverage for many of them. The site also gives the visitor useful nursing links in a separate section. One of the best things at this site is a recording of Florence Nightingale from 1890. You can actually listen to her voice!

Contact: internurse@internurse.com

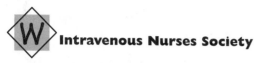 **Intravenous Nurses Society**

www.ins1.org

The Intravenous Nurses Society (INS) is a national, nonprofit membership organization formed in 1973. Membership is open to all healthcare professionals from all practice settings involved or interested in the specialty practice of intravenous nursing. INS is dedicated to advancing the delivery of quality intravenous therapy through stringent standards of practice and professional ethics, and promoting research and education in the intravenous specialty.

Contact: Chris.Hunt@ins1.org

 ITD-JNL

listserv@maelstrom.stjohns.edu

Electronic distribution of the *Information and Technology for the Disabled Journal*. On subscribing, you will asked to confirm your intention of joining the list.

Subscribe ITD-JNL Firstname Lastname

 ITNA

listserv@listserv.bcm.tmc.edu

Discussion list for the International TeleNurses Association. On subscribing, you will asked to confirm your intention of joining the list.

Subscribe ITNA Firstname Lastname

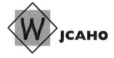 **JCAHO**

www.jcaho.org

This Website, from the Joint Commission on Accreditation of Healthcare Organizations, is designed to inform the healthcare community and the public about the Joint Commission, its services, and its products. Information is updated regularly to reflect the ongoing changes in health. The Quality Calendar has a new quality quote every day.

Contact: webmaster@jcaho.org

JEFFLINE at Thomas Jefferson University

http://Jeffline.tju.edu/

JEFFLINE is the entry point to Thomas Jefferson University WWW information service. The clever interface—it looks like an office—directs you to points of interest. For example, the books on the shelf take you to the library, the calendar on the bulletin board takes you to current events, and the lab coat on the hook in the corner takes you to patient care resources.

Contact: help@jeffline.tju.edu

 Johns Hopkins University School of Nursing

www.son.jhmi.edu

Information on the school of nursing, the faculty, courses, and programs. Within the Center for Nursing Research is a useful document with tips on writing a successful grant application.

Contact: websugg@son.jhmi.edu

 Journal of Neonatal Nursing

www.bizjet.com/jnn/

The *Journal of Neonatal Nursing* is the official journal of the UK Neonatal Nurses Association and the journal for professionals who care for neonates and their families. Included are abstracts of all the articles published in the current issue of the journal. Full text articles are available for a fee.

Contact: jnn@bizjet.com

 Judy Norris' Home Page

www.ualberta.ca/~jrnorris/

Judy Norris' Website contains the QualPage, resources related to qualitative research; research studies; a nursing theory page with extensive information and links; the Canadian Association for the History of Nursing page; and the NURSENET Page, resources for the NURSENET Listserv subscribers.

Contact: Judy Norris, Judy.Norris@ualberta.ca

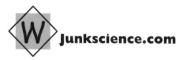 **Junkscience.com**

www.junkscience.com

"All the junk that's fit to debunk." Steven J. Milloy publishes Junkscience.com and is an adjunct scholar at the Cato Institute.

Contact: e-mail directly from the site

 Juvenile Diabetes Foundation International (JDF)— The Diabetes Research Foundation

www.jdfcure.org

JDF's main objective is to support and fund research to find a cure for diabetes and its complications. JDF's site offers diabetes information and news updates, research, and membership information. Fact sheets, research initiatives, publications and information about local chapters are available.

Contact: info@jdfcure.org

 Kent State University School of Nursing

www.kent.edu/nursing/

Kent State University School of Nursing was established in 1967. It offers one of the most comprehensive programs of study in nursing in Ohio. It is the largest school of nursing in Ohio and ranks in the 98th percentile in size in the United States. The school enjoys a reputation for excellent academic performance, clinical knowledge, and leadership abilities of its students and graduates. This site is also the home for the *Online Journal of Issues in Nursing*.

Contact: nursing@kent.edu

 Knowledge Base: Online Research Methods Textbook

http://trochim.human.cornell.edu/kb/index.htm

The Research Methods Knowledge Base is a comprehensive Web-based textbook that addresses all of the topics in a typical introductory undergraduate or graduate course in social research methods. It covers the entire research process, including formulating research questions; sampling (probability and nonprobability); measurement (surveys, scaling, qualitative, unobtrusive); research design (experimental and quasi-experimental); data analysis; and, writing the research paper. It also addresses the major theoretical and philosophical underpinnings of research, including the idea of validity in research; reliability of measures; and ethics. The Knowledge Base was designed to be different from the many typical research methods texts. It uses an informal, conversational style to engage both the newcomer and the more experienced student of research. Be sure to check out the decision matrix at http://trochim.human.cornell.edu/ojtrial/ojhome.htm to learn more about Type I and Type II errors. Developed by William Trochim at Cornell University.

Contact: William Trochim, wmt1@cornell.edu

 Latex Allergy Links

http://pw2.netcom.com/~nam1/latex_allergy.html

A comprehensive site on latex allergy and related links throughout the Internet.

Contact: Nancy A. Mitchell, latexallergy@ix.netcom.com

 LearnWell RN Online

www.learnwell.org/

Learnwell Resources, Inc. is a California nonprofit corporation with continuing education courses on health and ethics for CE credit. E-mail or fax your completed test to receive credit.

Contact: R. Klimes, PhD, edu@learnwell.org

 License to Care

www.nurseid.com

This Website acts as a sounding board for the nursing community. Share your stories, frustrations, and hopes. They promote the licensed nurse in the age of managed care, downsizing, and deskilling. You can order the RN and LPN lapel pins worn on ER and Chicago Hope at this site.

Contact: buzzbeat@aol.com

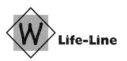 **Life-Line**

www.life-line.org/health/index.html

Informative consumer site on health insurance by the Life and Health Insurance Foundation for Education. Includes information on the Canadian health insurance system as well as the U.S. system.

Contact: webmaster@life-line.org or e-mail directly from the site

 Lippincott Williams & Wilkins Publishers

www.lww.com

Lippincott Williams & Wilkins is a world leader in information resources for nursing, medical, and allied health professionals and students. For over 200 years, the Lippincott name has become synonymous with nursing education for students, faculty, and practicing nurses. Texts explore modern nursing issues such as healthcare reform, community-based practice, patient and family teaching, cultural diversity, and others. Lippincott Williams & Wilkins is a multimedia company. In addition to textbooks, the Lippincott nursing imprint publishes journals, videos, audiocassettes, interactive video discs, and CD-ROMS, offering students new and valuable ways to learn. Lippincott is the publisher of *Computers in Nursing*, the only journal dedicated to nursing informatics.

Contact: webmaster@lww.com

 Liszt

www.liszt.com

If you are looking for a mailing list, check Liszt. This searchable database includes more than 90,000 mailing lists, with descriptions and subscription information.

Contact: liszt@liszt.com

LNCNURSE

LNCNURSE@ontosystems.com

A discussion group for legal nurse consultants. On subscribing, you will be asked to e-mail the list owner with some information about yourself and the reason you wish to join the list.

Type "subscribe" (no quotes) in the subject line of the message.

London Health Sciences Centre

http://www.lhsc.on.ca/

Clinical or critical pathways are a patient management tool that support continuous quality improvement, efficient resource utilization, and quality patient care. The development of clinical pathways at London Health Sciences Centre was driven by several key goals: to decrease resources and increase healthcare demands; to maintain high quality, patient-centered care; and to reduce length of stay. A starter kit for implementing clinical pathways has been developed by the center to assist patient care teams and healthcare organizations embarking on the task of developing clinical pathways, and is available for purchase.

Contact: webmaster@lhsc.on.ca

Lupus Foundation of America

www.lupus.org

The mission of the Lupus Foundation of America is to educate and support those affected by lupus and to find the cure. The "Living With Lupus" Website strives to contribute to the accomplishment of this mission by providing those within the Internet community who are affected by lupus a source of up-to-date information and support.

Contact: e-mail directly from the site

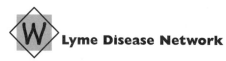

Lyme Disease Network

http://www.lymenet.org

The Lyme Disease Network is a nonprofit foundation dedicated to public education of the prevention and treatment of Lyme disease and other tick-borne illnesses.

Contact: Bill Stolow, bill@LymeNet.org

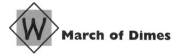

March of Dimes

www.modimes.org

Four major problems threaten the health of America's babies: birth defects, infant mortality, low birthweight, and lack of prenatal care. The March of Dimes has adopted goals for the year 2000 to bring us closer to the day when all babies will be born healthy. The Website defines those goals and includes information on research initiatives, a health library, programs, and public affairs.

Contact: e-mail directly from the site

 Massachusetts General Hospital

www.mgh.harvard.edu

Massachusetts General Hospital's Website contains extensive health-related resources. Departmental pages offer disease-specific information and links for patients and health professionals.

Contact: webmaster@mgh.harvard.edu

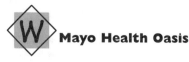

Mayo Health Oasis

www.mayohealth.org

A multifaceted online health information service sponsored by the Mayo Clinic. There are articles on allergies, Alzheimer's disease, cancer, diet and nutrition, cardiac disease, women's health, and more. A helpful search feature allows you to find resources of interest easily.

Contact: e-mail directly from the site

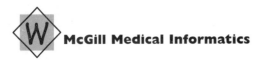 **McGill Medical Informatics**

www.mmi.mcgill.ca

A site with a wide variety of medical informatics links and information, including the National Digital Library and a Canada-wide image database for medical teaching and learning.

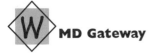 **MD Gateway**

www.mdgateway.com

MD Gateway is an Internet on-ramp for busy clinicians, to help direct them to information on the Internet that will help them care for their patients efficiently and assist them in operating their practices. Its purpose is to help busy clinicians keep abreast of medical developments, update them on professional issues that affect them, and assist them in running their practices efficiently while complying with Medicare rules.

 Medical College of Georgia School of Nursing

www.mcg.edu/son/

A stop here will deliver information about the school's academic programs, faculty, departments, curriculum, and research efforts. There are also links to other resources within the school.

Contact: Brenda Maddox, bmaddox@mail.mcg.edu

 Medical Informatics Laboratory

http://ipvaimed9.unipv.it/

Website of the Medical Informatics Laboratory at the University of Pavia, Italy. Includes descriptions of ongoing research projects in knowledge-based systems and artificial intelligence.

Contact: clara@aim.unipv.it

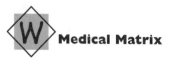 **Medical Matrix**

www.medmatrix.org

Ranked, peer-reviewed, annotated, and updated clinical medicine resources. An extremely comprehensive listing can be found at this site. It does require free registration.

Contact: Gary Malet, MD, gmalet@medmatrix.org

 Medical Records Institute (MRI)

www.medrecinst.com

MRI works to promote the development and acceptance of electronic health records, to support the industry and developers in their efforts, to educate providers about their options in migrating toward electronic health record systems, and to provide information to other parties involved in the process. MRI communicates this message through newsletters, publications, seminars, conferences, symposia, and developers' programs, as well as by participating in applied research and standards work in select areas of interest.

Contact: Jason Glass, jasong@medrecinst.com

 Medicine Planet

www.medicineplanet.com

Medicine Planet, Inc. is dedicated to providing travelers worldwide with definitive, one-stop health resources before, during and after a journey. With this goal in mind, a team of travel medicine experts provides a comprehensive offering of health information, products, tools and services on the Web.

Contact: info@medicineplanet.com

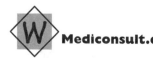 **Mediconsult.com**

www.mediconsult.com

Mediconsult.com is a "virtual medical center," providing quality, patient-oriented medical information and moderated support to patients, families, and healthcare professionals. Its mission is to provide timely, comprehensive, and accessible medical information on chronic medical conditions, using the latest available technology to deliver information efficiently. Access to the site is free.

Contact: information@mediconsult.com

 MED-JOKES

Majordomo@list.pitt.edu

Medical humor and jokes. Can be crude—do not subscribe if you are easily offended. The list runs on the Majordomo system. On subscribing, you will be asked to confirm your intention of joining the list.

Subscribe MED-JOKES

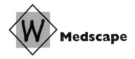 **Medscape**

www.medscape.com

Medscape offers specialists, primary care physicians, and other health professionals a robust and integrated multispecialty medical information and education tool. You may choose a personal Medscape home page from an assortment of specialty sites, primary care medicine sites, and nonclinical sites such as "Money & Medicine" or "Humor & Medicine." After a one-time free registration, Medscape automatically delivers to you the site you specify or that best fits your profile. Medscape is built around practice-oriented content. Each specialty site pools, filters, and delivers pertinent updated content from tens of thousands of medical journal articles, expert-authored state-of-the-art surveys in disease management, Next-Day Summaries from major medical meetings, and more.

Contact: webmaster@mail.medscape.com

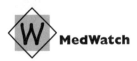 **MedWatch**

www.fda.gov/medwatch/

MedWatch, the FDA Medical Products Reporting Program, is an initiative designed both to educate all health professionals about the critical importance of being aware of, monitoring for, and reporting adverse events and problems to FDA and/or the manufacturer, and to ensure that new safety information is rapidly communicated to the medical community, thereby improving patient care. The MedWatch program is supported by over 140 organizations, representing health professionals and industry that have signed on as MedWatch Partners to help achieve these goals.

Contact: e-mail directly from the site

 Men in American Nursing History

www.geocities.com/Athens/Forum/6011/

A slide show that tells the story of men in American nursing history.

Contact: Bruce Wilson, wilson@hiline.net

 MENOPAUS

listserv@maelstrom.stjohns.edu

Discussion list on menopause and related women's issues. The list runs on the Listserv system. On subscribing, you will be asked to confirm your intention of joining the list.

Subscribe MENOPAUS Firstname Lastname

 Mental Health InfoSource

www.mhsource.com

An online community for mental health, this site includes patient and professional information, news, continuing education, and consultation.

Contact: Heather Orey, webmaster@mhsource.com

 Mental Health Net

http://mentalhelp.net/

Mental Health Net (MHN) was created in September 1995, as a free service to the worldwide mental health community of professionals and laypeople. It includes thousands of resources, and it covers disorders such as depression, anxiety, and chronic fatigue syndrome, to professional issues on psychiatry, psychology, and social work.

Contact: Mark Dombeck, PhD, mark@cmhc.com

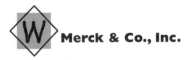 **Merck & Co., Inc.**

www.merck.com

Merck's Website gives an overview of the pharmaceutical company's major divisions, annual reports, FAQs, research, and product information. One particularly useful feature at this site is the classic *Merck Manual of Diagnosis and Treatment*. The entire manual is online and can be easily searched.

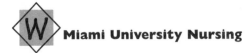 **Miami University Nursing**

www.sas.muohio.edu/nsg/

This Website from the Department of Nursing at Miami University in Ohio has information about its programs, faculty, and courses.

Contact: info@eas.muohio.edu

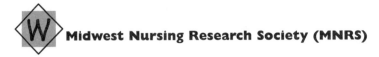 **Midwest Nursing Research Society (MNRS)**

www.mnrs.org

The Midwest Nursing Research Society is an organization devoted to the promotion, dissemination, and utilization of nursing research in all healthcare service and educational settings throughout the 13-state region of the Midwest. The MNRS Website provides information on nursing research, funding sources, publications, program meetings, and information about the MNRS.

Contact: info@mnrs.org

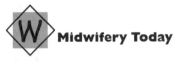 **Midwifery Today**

www.midwiferytoday.com

Through networking and education, Midwifery Today's mission is to return midwifery care to its rightful position in the family; to make midwifery care the norm throughout the world; and to redefine midwifery as a vital partnership with women. Information on publications, educational materials, and conferences sponsored by Midwifery Today. The site includes information for authors and full text of selected articles, as well as *The Birthkit Newsletter*.

Contact: inquiries@midwiferytoday.com

Morbidity and Mortality Weekly Report

http://www2.cdc.gov/mmwr

The *Morbidity and Mortality Weekly Report* (*MMWR*) Series is prepared by the Centers for Disease Control and Prevention (CDC). The data in the weekly *MMWR* are provisional, based on weekly reports to CDC by state health departments. The reporting week concludes at close of business on Friday; compiled data on a national basis are officially released to the public on the succeeding Friday. Free e-mail subscriptions to *MMWR* are available at the site.

Contact: mmwrq@cdc.gov

 Mosby, Inc.

www.mosby.com

Mosby, a Harcourt Health Sciences Company, is a publisher of books, journals, and serial publications in the health sciences (e.g., medicine, nursing, allied health sciences, dentistry, veterinary medicine) and selected college disciplines (e.g., health, physical education and recreation, nutrition, and chemistry). Mosby's Web page contains catalogs, customer support, conference and seminar updates, and online services.

Contact: e-mail directly from the site

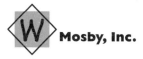 **MS Direct: Multiple Sclerosis Discussion**

http://dean.sporleder.aquila.com

A discussion group on multiple sclerosis. In his introduction to the page, Dean Sporleder writes, "I started this in august 1995 when a person close to me was diagnosed with ms, I have found it helps me work through some things and helps others find their way around ms resources on the Internet."

Contact: Dean Sporleder, msdirect@aquila.com

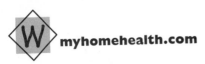

myhomehealth.com

www.myhomehealth.com

From the publishers of home health line, this Website features breaking news in home health care, as well as resources, links, and a discussion list.

Contact: customerrelations@myhomehealth.com

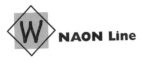

NAON Line

http://naon.inurse.com/

Website of the National Association of Orthopedic Nurses. News, events, education, certification information, and an online forum are featured.

Contact: naon@ajj.com

National Alliance for the Mentally Ill

www.nami.org

The National Alliance for the Mentally Ill (NAMI) Website offers extensive information about mental illness. With more than 210,000 members, NAMI is the nation's leading grassroots advocacy organization solely dedicated to improving the lives of persons with severe mental illnesses, including schizophrenia, bipolar disorder (manic-depressive illness), major depression, obsessive-compulsive disorder, and severe anxiety disorders.

Contact: webteam@www.nami.org

National Alliance of Breast Cancer Organizations

www.nabco.org

NABCO is the leading nonprofit central resource for information about breast cancer and a network of more than 375 organizations that provide detection, treatment and care to hundreds of thousands of American women. This site provides current information about breast cancer, updates on breast cancer–related events, clinical trials, support groups, and NABCO News.

Contact: NABCOinfo@aol.com

National Association for Home Care

www.nahc.org

Virtual headquarters of the National Association for Home Care, with information on legislation and regulatory issues, facts about home care, membership, meetings, conferences, and news. Includes a listing of state associations and a home care and hospice locator.

Contact: webmaster@nahc.org

 ## National Association of Associate Degree Nursing

www.noadn.org

Website of N-OADN, the leading advocate for associate degree nursing education practice. The association promotes collaboration in charting the future of healthcare education and delivery.

Contact: noadn@noadn.org

 ## National Association of Neonatal Nurses

www.nann.org

Website of the National Association of Neonatal Nurses, the association specifically for nurses practicing in this specialty.

Contact: info@nann.org

 ## National Association of Pediatric Nurse Associates and Practitioners

www.napnap.org

NAPNAP is the professional organization that advocates for children (infants through young adults) and provides leadership for Pediatric Nurse Practitioners who deliver Primary care in a variety of settings. The Website offers news, legislative information, products and services, and membership information.

Contact: info@napnap.org

National Association of School Nurses, Inc.

www.nasn.org

Website of the National Association of School Nurses, Inc., with information on the organization, membership, conferences, and materials available for purchase.

Contact: nasn@nasn.org

 National Ataxia Foundation

www.ataxia.org

The National Ataxia Foundation is a nonprofit organization established in 1957 with the primary mission of encouraging and supporting research into hereditary ataxia, a group of chronic and progressive neurologic disorders affecting coordination. There are more than 45 affiliated chapters and support groups throughout the United States and Canada. This page lists chapter contact information, upcoming events, publications, and support groups.

Contact: NAF@ataxia.org

 National Black Nurses Association

www.nbna.org

The National Black Nurses Association, Inc. (NBNA) is a professional nursing organization representing more than 150,000 African-American nurses throughout the United States. NBNA's mission is to provide a forum for collective action by nurses to investigate, define, and advocate for the healthcare needs of African Americans and to implement strategies that ensure access to health care, equal to, or above healthcare standards of the larger society. NBNA is committed to improving the quality of life of persons who share the African-American heritage and other ethnic groups.

Contact: nbna@erols.com

National Clearinghouse for Alcohol and Drug Information (NCADI)

www.health.org

This Website is a service of the Center for Substance Abuse Prevention, Substance Abuse and Mental Health Services Administration, U.S. Public Health Service, and the U.S. Department of Health and Human Services. Visitors will find news, referrals, publications, statistics, forums, databases, a calendar of events, related links, and information about NCADI. The Girl Power section seeks to reinforce and sustain these positive values among girls ages 9 to 14 by targeting health messages to the unique needs, interests, and challenges of girls.

Contact: webmaster@health.org

 National Council of State Boards of Nursing

www.ncsbn.org

This Website was created by the NCLEX people. News, information, and links to state boards of nursing.

Contact: info@ncsbn.org

 National Guideline Clearinghouse

www.ngc.gov

The National Guideline Clearinghouse (NGC) is a public resource for evidence-based clinical practice guidelines. NGC is sponsored by the Agency for Healthcare Research and Quality (AHRQ) in partnership with the American Medical Association and the American Association of Health Plans.

Contact: info@guideline.gov

 National Health Information Center (NHIC)

http://nhic-nt.health.org

The NHIC is a health information referral service that puts health professionals and consumers who have health questions in touch with those organizations that are best able to provide answers. NHIC was established in 1979 by the Office of Disease Prevention and Health Promotion (ODPHP), Office of Public

Health and Science, Office of the Secretary, U.S. Department of Health and Human Services. The NHIC Health Information Resource Database includes 1,100 organizations and government offices that provide health information on request. Entries include contact information, short abstracts, and information about publications and services that the organizations provide.

Contact: NHICinfo@health.org

 National Hospice and Palliative Care Organization

www.nhpco.org

The National Hospice and Palliative Care Organization is committed to improving end-of-life care and expanding access to hospice care with the goal of profoundly enhancing quality of life for people dying in America and their loved ones. This site has information about the organization, membership, and locations of hospices throughout the United States.

Contact: helpline@nhpco.org

 National Institute of Allergy and Infectious Disease (NIAID)

www.niaid.nih.gov

NIAID provides the major support for scientists conducting research aimed at developing better ways to diagnose, treat, and prevent the many infectious, immunologic, and allergic diseases that afflict people worldwide. The Website has links to the most up-to-date information resources, as well as research and reference tools.

Contact: e-mail directly from the site

 National Institute of Diabetes and Digestive and Kidney Diseases (NIDDK)

www.niddk.nih.gov

The National Institute of Diabetes and Digestive and Kidney Diseases (NIDDK) is part of the National Institutes of Health. NIDDK conducts and supports research on many of the most serious diseases affecting public health. The Institute supports much of the clinical research on the diseases of internal medicine and related subspecialty fields, as well as many basic science disciplines.

Contact: Kathy Kranzfelder, kathy_kranzfelder@nih.gov

 ## National Institute of Neurological Disorders and Stroke (NINDS)

www.ninds.nih.gov

NINDS, an agency of the federal government and a component of the National Institutes of Health and the U.S. Public Health Service, is a lead agency for the congressionally designated Decade of the Brain and the leading supporter of biomedical research on disorders of the brain and nervous system. A stop here will render general information on neurological disorders, a link to available publications, and a database of voluntary health agency contact information.

Contact: e-mail directly from the site

 ## National Institute of Nursing Research (NINR)

www.nih.gov/ninr/

NINR's mission is to promote science that strengthens nursing practice and improves health care. NINR supports interdisciplinary research and research training in universities, hospitals, and research centers across the country and conducts intramural investigations at NIH. There are links to extensive information on research funding and programs, as well as contact information for the NINR's major areas of concentration. The site also has a useful link to schools of nursing throughout the United States, organized by state.

Contact: info@ninr.nih.gov

 ## National Institute of Occupational Safety and Health

www.cdc.gov/niosh/

NIOSH is part of the Centers for Disease Control and Prevention (CDC) and is the only federal Institute responsible for conducting research and making recommendations for the prevention of work-related illnesses and injuries. Although NIOSH and OSHA were created by the same Act of Congress, they are two distinct agencies with separate responsibilities. OSHA is in the Department of Labor and is responsible for creating and enforcing workplace safety and health regulations. NIOSH is in the Department of Health and Human Services and is a research agency. This Website has been established to provide information about NIOSH and related activities. From these pages you are able to walk inside NIOSH, by subject or category, and find information and services. There are numerous health and safety publications, in both English and Spanish.

Contact: e-mail directly from the site

 ## National Institutes of Health (NIH)

www.nih.gov

Any Internet-traveling health professional should plan a stop at the NIH Web-site. The NIH Website offers news and events; health information; grants and contracts; scientific resources; and links to other institutes and offices, including the National Institute of Nursing Research and the W.G. Magnuson Clinical Center Nursing Department. NIH is a good all-around resource for nurses from all specialties.

Contact: nihinfo@od.nih.gov

 ## National Institutes of Health: Warren Grant Magnuson Clinical Center Nursing Department

www.cc.nih.gov/nursing/

For a complete listing of National Institutes of Health resources, start your journey at www.nih.gov. For a more nursing-specific list of resources, the nursing department page has links to nursing and health-related Websites maintained by universities, the Centers for Disease Control and Prevention, and the National Institute of Nursing Research. There are also links to federal resources, Internet search engines, and other useful resources.

Contact: bbrown@nih.gov

 ## National League for Nursing

www.nln.org

This site is a resource center for nursing education, practice, and research. Here you will find features offering you the latest information about NLN membership, Constituent Leagues, accreditation, testing services and tests, and meetings and workshops.

Contact: nlnweb@nln.org

National Library of Medicine

www.nlm.nih.gov

The National Library of Medicine is the world's largest medical library. Every significant program of the library is represented on this site, from medical history to biotechnology. Visitors here will find news, information about NLM, and its services. Users can access NLM databases and publications and keep up to date on research activities, grants, and contracts.

 National Multiple Sclerosis Society (NMSS)

www.nmss.org

NMSS is dedicated to advancing the cure, prevention, and treatment of multiple sclerosis and to improving the lives of those affected by the disease. Visitors to the NMSS site will find information on multiple sclerosis, resources, NMSS, and local chapters, and opportunities to get involved.

Contact: info@nmss.org

 National Network of Libraries of Medicine (NN/LM)

www.nnlm.nlm.nih.gov

Start at the NN/LM for program and resource notes, health-related federal agencies, and other health links. Search NN/LM, accessing resources for medical librarians by U.S. region and research funding resources, and connect to Internet GratefulMed and PubMed. An archive of JCAHO survey reports is available at the site.

Contact: e-mail directly from the site

 National Neurofibromatosis Foundation

www.nf.org

The National Neurofibromatosis Foundation, Inc. has detailed information on Type 1 and Type 2 of the genetic disorder neurofibromatosis as well as schwannomatosis. Major headings introduce a set of information for patients and one for healthcare professionals. The patient information covers the basic issues of the symptoms, diagnosis, and genetics of neurofibromatosis. The section for healthcare professionals covers the more technical issues, such as molecular biology, mode of inheritance, and diagnostic criteria. This page also has information on support groups, online resources, and an overview of the National Neurofibromatosis Foundation.

Contact: nnff@nf.org

 ## National Rehabilitation Information Center (NARIC)

www.naric.com

NARIC is a library and information center covering disability and rehabilitation. Funded by the National Institute on Disability and Rehabilitation Research (NIDRR), NARIC collects and disseminates the results of federally funded research projects. The collection, which also includes commercially published books, journal articles, and audiovisuals, grows at a rate of 300 documents a month. NARIC has more than 60,000 documents on all aspects of disability rehabilitation.

Contact: jchaiken@kra.com

 ## National Rosacea Society

www.rosacea.org

Website for the National Rosacea Society, with information on this condition, educational materials, and other resources.

Contact: rosaceas@aol.com

 ## National Stroke Association (NSA)

www.stroke.org

National Stroke Association's mission is to reduce the incidence and impact of stroke by changing the way stroke is viewed and treated. NSA is a leading national organization dedicating 100% of its resources and efforts toward stroke through prevention, treatment, rehabilitation, research, and support for stroke survivors and their families. NSA's Website lists educational offerings, facts about and risks associated with stroke, membership information, and volunteer opportunities.

Contact: e-mail directly from the site

National Women's Health Information Center

www.4woman.gov

The National Women's Health Information Center (NWHIC) is a one-stop gateway for women seeking health information. A service of the Office on Women's Health in the U.S. Department of Health and Human Services, NWHIC is a free information and resource service on women's health issues for consumers, healthcare professionals, researchers, educators, and students. The bilingual (English/Spanish) site is fully searchable and contains a wealth of information on health issues for women. All of the information is free of copyright restrictions and may be copied for personal or patient information.

Contact: 4woman@soza.com

 ## Nell Hodgson Woodruff School of Nursing

www.nurse.emory.edu

The Nell Hodgson Woodruff School of Nursing is the professional collegiate nursing school of Emory University in Atlanta, Georgia, and is one of seven divisions constituting the Robert W. Woodruff Health Sciences Center. A visitor here will find the school's mission; goals; and information on the academic programs, faculty, and enrollment.

Contact: e-mail directly from the site

 ## NEONATAL-TALK

neonatal-talk@liststar.bizjet.com

Discussion list for nurses and health professionals in neonatal care. On submitting a request to join the list, you will be automatically added to the list.

To subscribe, send a message to the above address with the word "subscribe" (no quotes) in the subject line. Leave the body of the message blank.

Neurosciences on the Internet

www.neuroguide.com

Neurosciences on the Internet contains a searchable index of neuroscience resources available on the Web and other parts of the Internet. Neurobiology, neurology, neurosurgery, psychiatry, psychology, cognitive science sites, and information on human neurological diseases are covered. Check out the Best Bets page for some excellent links.

Contact: Neil A. Busis, nab@neuroguide.com

 Neurosurgery Teaching Files

www.neuro.upstate.edu/neuro/teachfile/

Tutorial on how to take a history, anatomy review, common neurologic emergencies, and more, all presented by the Department of Neurosurgery at Syracuse University.

Contact: neurosrg@upstate.edu

 New England Journal of Medicine

www.nejm.org

The New England Journal of Medicine offers abstracts of Original Articles (reports of original clinical research) and Special Articles (reports of research on health policy) online without charge, as well as several methods of searching for articles. Subscribers to the print journal may access the full text of the journal online.

Contact: comments@nejm.org

 New York State Department of Health

www.health.state.ny.us

The New York State Department of Health Website is divided into the following categories: From the Commissioner page; directory services; how to get New York State vital records information; information for consumers; information for physicians and other healthcare providers; healthcare data for researchers; and a public health forum. A " What's New" page highlights recent postings. Also included are links to the Department's Wadsworth Center, the School of Public Health, Health Research, Inc., the NYS Partnership for Long-Term Care, Helen Hayes Hospital, Roswell Park Cancer Institute, the Task Force on Life and the Law, as well as links to other New York State government resources and health-related sites.

Contact: nyhealth@health.state.ny.us

 New York State Nurses' Association

www.nysna.org

Website of the New York State Nurses' Association, with membership information, continuing education, economic and general nursing news, governmental affairs, and more.

Contact: info@nysna.org

 New York University Division of Nursing

www.nyu.edu/education/nursing/

This Website has information on the academic programs, faculty, research programs, and continuing education. There are also nursing links and a pointer to special announcements.

Contact: Anthony Rini, anthony.rini@nyu.edu

 NicNet: The Nicotine and Tobacco Network

www.nicnet.org

An index to smoking resources on the Internet, maintained by the Arizona Program for Nicotine and Tobacco Research. Includes life-saving information, monthly features, and the latest trends in research.

Contact: nicnet@w3.arizona.edu

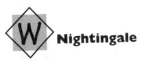 Nightingale

http://nightingale.con.utk.edu/

This is a Website located at the University of Tennessee, Knoxville College of Nursing. Nightingale was one of the first Internet offerings that focused on nursing. Information about the school, its programs, faculty, and research is available at the site.

Contact: nightingale@cn.gw.utk.edu

 NIH-Guide to Grants and Contracts Database

www.grants.nih.gov/grants/guide/

The NIH guide is available weekly. This site provides a searchable archive of the complete NIH Guide to grants and contracts. It is also possible to browse each weekly issue of the Guide at this site.

Contact: grantsinfo@nih.gov

 NOAH: New York Online Access to Health

www.noah.cuny.edu

New York Online Access to Health (NOAH) is your guide in Spanish and English to the latest health information and resources from volunteer and local governmental agencies, and from other health sites on the Internet. NOAH has information on a wide variety of topics, including aging, AIDS, alternative medicine, cancer, diabetes, healthy living, heart disease and stroke, nutrition, personal health, pregnancy, sexuality, sexually transmitted diseases, and tuberculosis. There is also patient information and a listing of healthcare organizations in New York state.

Contact: webmaster@noah.cuny.edu

NP-Clinical

Majordomo@nurse.net

Clinical practice issues for nurse practitioners. Nonclinical issues can be discussed on NPINFO. The list runs on the Majordomo system. On subscribing, you will be asked to confirm your intention of joining the list.

Subscribe NP-Clinical Your e-mail address

 NPINFO

Majordomo@nurse.net

Discussion list for nurse practitioners. The list runs on the Majordomo system. On subscribing, you will be asked to confirm your intention of joining the list.

Subscribe NPINFO Your e-mail address

 NP-Students

Majordomo@nurse.net

Discussion list among nurse practitioner students, newly graduated nurse practitioners, and nurse practitioner mentors and faculty. The list runs on the Majordomo system. On subscribing, you will be asked to confirm your intention of joining the list.

Subscribe NP-Students Your e-mail address

 NRSINGED

listserv@listserv.louisville.edu

Discussion list on nursing education, primarily for educators. The list runs on the Listserv system. On subscribing, you will be asked to confirm your intention of joining the list.

Subscribe NRSINGED Firstname Lastname

NRSING-L

http://mailman.amia.org/listinfo/nursing-l

Discussion list on nursing informatics. To join, go to the Website listed earlier, where a form will navigate you through the subscription process.

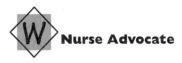 **Nurse Advocate**

www.nurseadvocate.org

"Dedicated to the recognition and resolution of workplace violence experienced by nurses; in support of those who have experienced violence; and in memory of those who have died." A discussion list is available for subscription at the site.

Contact: Carrie Lybecker, RN, carriejl@home.com

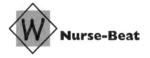 **Nurse-Beat**

www.nurse-beat.com

Online cardiac nursing journal, with ECG strip interpretation, cardiac pharmacology, and more.

Contact: Debra Kumar, RN, BSN, CCRN, editor@nurse-beat.com

 NurseLRC

Majordomo@douglas.bc.ca

Discussion list for nursing Learning Resource Center faculty and staff to network about psychomotor skill acquisition, care and maintenance of equipment, instructional strategies, computer and audiovisual resources, and funding sources. The list runs on the Majordomo system. You will be automatically added to the list when you submit your request to join.

Subscribe NurseLRC (Note: do not include your name or e-mail address.)

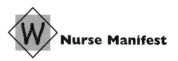 **Nurse Manifest**

http://www.nursemanifest.com/

Nurse Manifest is a "A Nursing Manifesto: A Call to Conscience and Action," designed to raise awareness, to inspire action, and to open for discussion issues that are vital to health care around the globe.

Contact: facilitators@nursemanifest.com

 NURSENET

listserv@listserv.utoronto.ca

A global forum for discussion of nursing issues, maintained by Judy Norris. The list runs on the Listserv system. On subscribing, you will be asked to confirm your intention of joining the list.

Subscribe NURSENET Firstname Lastname

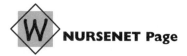 **NURSENET Page**

www.ualberta.ca/~jrnorris/nursenet/nn.html

The NURSENET Page is designed to accompany the Listserv, NURSENET. Includes stats on NURSENET, archives of interesting NURSENET discussions, and educational resources about the Internet.

Contact: Judy Norris, RN, PhD, judy.norris@ualberta.ca

 NURSERES

listserv@listserv.kent.edu

Discussion list on nursing research and related issues. The list runs on the Listserv system. On subscribing, you will be asked to confirm your intention of joining the list.

Subscribe NURSERES Firstname Lastname

NURSE-ROGERS

mailbase@mailbase.ac.uk

A discussion list for nurses from around the world to enter into scholarly debate and discuss latest developments and significant issues related to Martha Rogers' conceptual system, the Science of Unitary Human Beings. The list runs on the mailbase system. On subscribing, you will be asked to confirm your intention of joining the list.

JOIN nurse-rogers Firstname Lastname

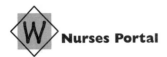 **Nurses Portal**

www.nursesportal.com

Formerly the Virtual Nurse site, a little bit of everything can be found at this site: chat rooms, message boards, funny nursing stories, and more.

Contact: webmaster@nursesportal.com

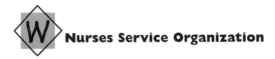 **Nurses Service Organization**

www.nso.com

Nurses Service Organization (NSO) is a provider of liability insurance for professional nurses. This site has information on their products. A free e-mail subscription to the *NSO Risk Advisor*, a newsletter with articles on legal and liability issues, is also available.

Contact: service@nso.com

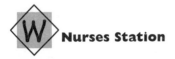 **Nurses Station**

www.nursesstationcatalog.com or www.nursesdirect.com

Gifts, scrubs, shoes, instruments, and more for sale online through this catalog vendor.

Contact: customerservice@nursesdirect.com

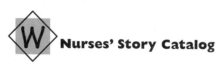

Nurses' Story Catalog

http://web.indstate.edu/nurs/nscat.htm

Nurses' Story Catalog is an Aesopic teaching assistant for nursing teachers, student nurses, nurses, and nurse researchers. Aesop, as you will recall, taught by telling stories that had points and wise sayings associated with them. This teaching method is in contrast to the Socratic method, taught by asking questions, and to the didactic or lecture method. Stories transmit information in a situation-specific framework, are easier to remember, pique interest in dry subject matter, operationalize general rules, and illustrate concrete applications of abstract principles. Nurses' Story Catalog, NSCat for short, is a computer program that stores and indexes a database of nursing stories. Teachers or students can search for stories by typing in key words. Julia M. Fine of the Indiana State University School of Nursing maintains this page. She welcomes submissions from nurses to add to her database of stories.

Contact: Julia M. Fine, nufine@befac.indstate.edu

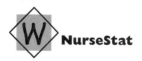

NurseStat

www.nursestat.com

"Welcome to NurseStat Online Services, the most comprehensive nursing Web community on the Internet. This is an effort of NurseStat, Inc. to allow nursing professionals one single locale for information, products and services. It is our sincere hope that we have created a site for nursing professionals where they can congregate, share ideas, access references, order products and services, advance their careers and education, investigate social, ethical and political topics affecting nursing or just plain chat."

Contact: Will Fowlkes, wfowlkes@sios.com

NURSE-UK

www.mailbase.ac.uk/lists/nurse-uk/

Discussion list for nurses in the United Kingdom. To join, go to the Website listed above, where a form will navigate you through the subscription process.

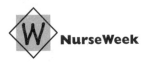 **NurseWeek**

www.nurseweek.com

NurseWeek is an online publication devoted to nursing. NurseWeek's mission is to support and promote the value of nursing by maintaining a forum for the exchange of information and ideas. The publication reports on local, regional, and national issues from a nursing perspective. It provides healthcare news, resources, and opportunities to help readers excel in their daily work and reach their career goals.

Contact: editor@nurseweek.com

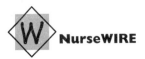 **NurseWIRE**

http://ideanurse.com/nursewire/

NurseWIRE is a service that lists nurse entrepreneurs and business opportunities on the Internet. As the Web becomes more available and widely used, more nurses in business will find it useful to "hang a shingle" here. Let these enterprising nurses know that you saw them on the Internet!

Contact: Peter Ramme, RN, peter@silicon.com

 Nursing and Health Care Resources on the Net

www.shef.ac.uk/~nhcon/

A comprehensive list of links for all aspects of nursing. Maintained by Rod Ward, a nurse in the United Kingdom; there is a wealth of international information available.

Contact: Rod Ward, Rod.Ward@Sheffield.ac.uk

 Nursing BCS Specialist Group

www.bcsnsg.org.uk

The Nursing Group of the British Computer Society contributes to national and international debates on information management and technology. The group seeks the views of members through focus groups and links with other bodies within the United Kingdom and with international bodies, such as the

International Nursing Informatics Society (INIS) and the European Federation for Medical Informatics (EFMI).

Contact: Rod Ward, rod.ward@sheffield.ac.uk

 Nursing: Caring for Those in Need

www.geocities.com/~nurse1/default.html

Website of Eric M. Zielinski, RN, BSN. Includes a feature of the month, interactive survey, the nurse's prayer, and more.

Contact: Eric M. Zielinski, RN, BSN, nurse1@geocities.com

 NursingCenter.com

www.nursingcenter.com

NursingCenter.com traces its origin to January 1995 when it debuted as AJN Online. It was recently relaunched as a nursing portal with greatly expanded content, personalization features and new payment methods for institutions. The Website now offers the tables of contents and abstracts of 24 journals. Many of these offer full text of feature articles for a fee. Over 300 hours of continuing education with instantaneous processing and certificates that print immediately can be purchased by entering a secure area and using a credit card. Group accounts that allow institutions to pay for CE and articles for their nurses is a new payment option. The Career Center, peer forums, and databases of organizations and certification have been expanded. Free Web e-mail and daily healthcare newsfeeds from Reuters have been added. Special personalization features allow the user to create a customized "My NursingCenter" with shortcuts to areas that the user frequents on the site. A File Drawer where CE and other purchased content can be stored and retrieved at any time provides another personal feature. A powerful new search engine makes finding information on the site quick and easy. The new MarketPlace provides opportunity for online shopping. Users who register on the site enjoy additional benefits and services; registration is free. Come see the new face of nursing at www.NursingCenter.com.

Contact: webmaster@nursingcenter.com

Nursing Center for Tobacco Intervention

www.con.ohio-state.edu/tobacco/

Nurses are effective providers of tobacco cessation interventions. The overall purpose of this site is to increase nurse provider participation in the delivery of tobacco cessation interventions with all tobacco users. Education, information, a forum for interchange, and information on timely topics are all available here.

Contact: ncti@osu.edu

 Nursing Editors On-Line

http://members.aol.com/suzannehj/naed.htm

This is an index of nursing journal and book editors. Query them online about your manuscript idea. The editors are listed alphabetically by the title of the journal they edit. You can scroll down, or you can use the "find" feature in your Web browser to locate the editors you want. Each e-mail address has a direct mail link, so all you need is one click on the e-mail address to link with an editor.

Contact: Suzanne Hall Johnson, suzannehj@aol.com

 Nursing Mothers' Association of Australia (NMAA)

http://avoca.vicnet.net.au/~nmaa/

The goal of the NMAA is to provide information for both breastfeeding women and for health professionals and others who are involved in supporting and promoting breastfeeding. Visitors here can find out more about this organization and access articles from the Lactation Resource Centre.

Contact: Jenny Gigacz, jenny@solcraft.com.au

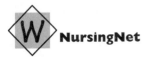 **NursingNet**

www.nursingnet.org

NursingNet was created to help further the knowledge and understanding of nursing for the public and to provide a forum for medical professionals and students to obtain and disseminate information about nursing and medically related subjects. This information includes, but is not limited to, student nursing, specialty nursing, healthcare issues, and insurance issues. NursingNet offers a chat room, an automated forum, links to other nursing-specific sites, and monthly features.

Contact: webmaster@nursingnet.org

 Nursing Ring

www.geocities.com/HotSprings/spa/3896/

If you have a Website devoted to nursing and want to get the word out to other nurses, consider joining the Nursing Ring. Details on how to do so are available at this site.

Contact: Kelly Gibbs, nurse@edesigns.org

 Nursing Standard Online

www.nursing-standard.co.uk/index.html

Nursing Standard Online archives articles and abstracts from *Nursing Standard*. Further details on the Royal College of Nursing, conferences, and continuing education opportunities are available at the site.

Contact: nursing.standard@rcn.org.uk

 Nursing Student WWW Page

www.csn.net/~tbracket/htm.htm

Information and resources for nursing students throughout the world.

Contact: Tim Brackett, Tim.Brackett@uchsc.edu

 Oakland University School of Nursing

www2.oakland.edu/nursing/

The School of Nursing at Oakland University offers undergraduate and graduate programs designed to prepare nurses to practice in the continuously changing healthcare system of today and tomorrow. This site includes general information about their programs. In addition, they are developing archives related to Dorothea E. Orem's Self-Care Deficit Theory of Nursing and Imogene King's Open Systems Model. Bibliographies of readings for both theories are available at this site.

Contact: nrsinfo@oakland.edu

 OB-GYN-L

listserv@obgyn.net

Professionally oriented discussion list for obstetrics, gynecology, and related issues. The list runs on the Listserv system. On subscribing, you will be automatically added to the list.

Subscribe OB-GYN-L Firstname Lastname

 Obsessive Compulsive Disorder Resource Center

www.ocdresource.com

The information on this site is offered to inform patients and healthcare professionals about obsessive-compulsive disorder (OCD)—what it is and what kind of medical treatment and emotional support is available. The site was created with input from OCD patients and medical experts. The site is sponsored by the Pharmacia & Upjohn Company and Solvay Pharmaceuticals.

 OCD (Obsessive Compulsive Disorders) Web Server

http://fairlite.com/ocd/

This obsessive-compulsive disorders (OCD) site is a good example of using the Web to create a community. Maintainers Mark and Kelly Luljak (Mark is an OCD sufferer) create an aura of compassion and optimism that is reflected in the postings to the OCD page's popular public bulletin board, the cornerstone of the site. The depth of the information resources available is also impressive; visitors will find personal narratives, medical articles, medication information, and links to other OCD-related sites on the Web.

Contact: webmaster@fairlite.com

OCD-L

listserv@vm.marist.edu

Discussion group on obsessive-compulsive disorder. The list runs on the Listserv system. On subscribing, you will be asked to confirm your intention of joining the list.

Subscribe OCD-L Firstname Lastname

 Ohio State University College of Nursing

www.con.ohio-state.edu/

Here a visitor will find general information, as well as nursing, medical, computing, and Internet resources. There are also pointers to the Health Science Colleges and the OSU Website. This site also links to the Nursing Center for Tobacco Intervention, which is affiliated with the college of nursing.

Contact: brownfield.3@osu.edu

 OHN-LIST

listserv@oise.utoronto.ca

Discussion list for occupational health nurses and allied professionals. On subscribing, you will be added to the list automatically.

Subscribe OHN-LIST

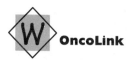 **OncoLink**

www.oncolink.upenn.edu

OncoLink was founded in 1994 by Penn cancer specialists with a mission to help cancer patients, families, healthcare professionals, and the general public get accurate cancer-related information at no charge. OncoLink is designed to make it easy for the general public to navigate through the pages and obtain the information. Through OncoLink you can get comprehensive information about specific types of cancer, updates on cancer treatments, and news about research advances. The information is updated everyday and provides information at various levels, from introductory to in-depth. If you are interested in learning about cancer, you will benefit from visiting OncoLink.

Contact: editors@oncolink.upenn.edu

 Oncology Nursing Society (ONS Online)

www.ons.org

ONS Online is a cancer information service for oncology nurses. Registration is required to access most areas of the site.

Contact: customer.service@ons.org

 Online Birth Center

www.moonlily.com/obc/

A comprehensive source of information on pregnancy, birth, and breastfeeding. The site includes articles, patient information, breastfeeding resources, lists of midwives, a parent's page, information on high-risk pregnancies, and more.

Contact: Donna Dolezal Zelzer, birth@moonlily.com

 Online Journal of Issues in Nursing

www.nursingworld.org/ojin/

The *Online Journal of Issues in Nursing* (*OJIN*) is a peer-reviewed publication that provides a forum for discussion of pertinent issues in nursing. *OJIN* defines an issue as a topic about which there are no right or wrong opinions but rather different viewpoints. The intent of this journal is to present different views on topics that affect nursing research, education, and practice, thus enabling readers to understand the full complexity of an issue. The interactive format of the journal encourages a dynamic dialogue, resulting in a comprehensive discussion of the topic, thereby building up the body of nursing knowledge and suggesting policy implications that enhance the health of the public.

Contact: ojin@kent.edu

On-Line Journal of Nursing Informatics

http://milkman.cac.psu.edu/~dxm12/OJNI.html

The aim of the *On-Line Journal of Nursing Informatics* (*OJNI*) is to publish peer-reviewed, original, high-quality scientific papers, review articles, practice-based articles, and databases related to nursing informatics.

Contact: Dee McGonigle PhD, RNC, FACCE, dxm12@psu.edu

 ## OVARIAN

listserv@listserv.acor.org

A discussion group devoted to ovarian cancer. The list runs on the Listserv system. On subscribing, you will be asked to confirm your intention of joining the list.

Subscribe OVARIAN Firstname Lastname

 ## Pain.com

www.pain.com

"A world of information on pain." Up-to-date information on pain, including JCAHO standards, educational modules, and a virtual library with thousands of full-text articles on pain and pain management.

Contact: editor@pain.com

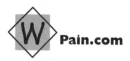 ## Pan American Health Organization

www.paho.org

This site presents information about the activities, publications, and services of the Pan American Health Organization, an international public health agency based in Washington, DC. The site includes news releases and the Country Health Profiles (an encyclopedia of the conditions and health concerns of every country in the Americas), databases, and library searches. The site is accessible in English or Spanish versions.

Contact: webmaster@paho.org

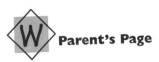 **Parent's Page**

www.efn.org/~djz/birth/babylist.html

This page is a resource for parents-to-be, as well as for parents of infants and small children. The Parent's Page is a good starting place for links to organizations, multimedia, mailing lists, and health resources that specialize in pregnancy and birth. There is also information about and connections to home-birth and midwifery resources, as well as adoption, family planning, infertility, and grief and loss.

Contact: Donna Dolezal Zelzer, birth@moonlily.com

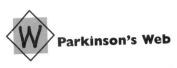 **Parkinson's Web**

http://pdweb.mgh.harvard.edu/

This Website contains a vast amount of information about Parkinson's disease and its treatment. It serves as a resource directory, pointing you to sources to information.

Contact: pdweb@cisco.com

 PARSE-L

listserv@listserv.utoronto.ca

Discussion group related to Parse's Theory of Human Becoming. The list runs on the Listserv system. Your request to join the list will be forwarded to the list owner for approval; once approved, you will be automatically added to the list.

Subscribe PARSE-L Firstname Lastname

 Pediatric Endocrinology Nursing Society

www.pens.org

Website for the Pediatric Endocrinology Nursing Society (PENS), with newsletter articles, conference information, membership resources, and more.

Contact: webmaster@pens.org

PEDIATRIC-PAIN

mailserv@ac.dal.ca

Pediatric pain discussion group. The list runs on the Mailserv system. On subscribing, you will be automatically added to the list.

Subscribe PEDIATRIC-PAIN Firstname Lastname

 Pediatric Points of Interest

www.med.jhu.edu/peds/neonatology/poi.html

Pediatric Points of Interest is a searchable collection of links to resources in Pediatrics and Child Health from the Department of Pediatrics and the Residency Program at Johns Hopkins University.

Contact: Christoph U. Lehmann, M.D., clehmann@welchlink.welch.jhu.edu

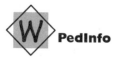 **PedInfo**

www.pedinfo.org

PedInfo: An Index of the Pediatric Internet is dedicated to the dissemination of online medical information for pediatricians and others interested in child health. There are many links to pediatric resources for parents, nurses, and physicians. There is a Web server search function, research resources, and subscription information for PEDS-INFORMATICS, a pediatric medical informatics mailing list.

Contact: webmaster@pedinfo.org

 PEDS-INFORMATICS

http://www.egroup.com/group/peds-informatics

Discussion group on pediatric medical informatics. Visit the Website listed above and follow the instructions to subscribe.

Pennsylvania State University School of Nursing

www.hhdev.psu.edu/nurs/nurs.htm

Information on the school of nursing at Penn State. There is a handy listing of faculty members and their research interests.

Contact: pxp10@psu.edu

 Perinatal Nursing Discussion List Webpage

http://wings.buffalo.edu/academic/department/nursing/mccartny/perintal.htm

Website to accompany the PNATALRN discussion group.

Contact: Patricia McCartney, mccartny@acsu.buffalo.edu

 PERIOP

Listproc@u.washington.edu

Discussion group for perioperative/OR/theatre nurses worldwide. The list runs on the Listproc system. On subscribing, you will be asked to confirm your intention of joining the list.

Subscribe PERIOP Firstname Lastname

 Pets and People: Companions in Therapy and Service

www.petsandpeople.org

Information on service dog training and animal-assisted therapy. Maintained by Pat Gonser, RN.

Contact: pandp@bigfoot.com

PharmInfoNet: Pharmaceutical Information Network

www.pharminfo.com

A comprehensive Website for pharmaceutical information. Major headings include articles, drug information, disease information, discussion groups, a glossary, PharmLinks, and the Gallery.

Contact: webmaster@pharminfo.com

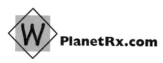 **PlanetRx.com**

www.planetrx.com

PlanetRx is one of several online pharmacies dispensing information about health conditions, along with prescription and over-the-counter medications. PlanetRx offerings include easy-to-read information on medical conditions, including conventional and alternative treatments, prevention, and self-care; information on prescription drugs, over-the-counter medications, vitamins, herbs, and other products; an online community: live chats and message boards for sharing ideas and information about health; Ask the Pharmacist, where staff pharmacists answer consumer questions privately, 24 hours a day; and personal services such as prescription refill reminders and warnings about drug interactions.

 Planned Parenthood

www.plannedparenthood.org

Website of the Planned Parenthood Federation of America, Inc. The site includes legislative updates, statistics, newsletters, and a library with information on contraception, abortion, parenting, and public affairs. A Spanish-language version is available at the site.

Contact: communications@ppfa.org

PNATALRN

listserv@listserv.acsu.buffalo.edu

Discussion group on perinatal nursing practice, education, and research.

Subscribe PNATALRN Firstname Lastname

 POLIO

listserv@maelstrom.stjohns.edu

Discussion group for persons affected by polio. Your request to join the list will be forwarded to the list owner for approval; after approval, you will be automatically added to the list.

Subscribe POLIO Firstname Lastname

 Polio Survivors Page

www.eskimo.com/~dempt/polio.html

This site is dedicated to persons affected by polio. Visitors will find listings of publications and newsletters on polio, support resources for the disabled, brief biographies of some polio survivors, and links to other polio WWW pages. The site is maintained by the Lincolnshire Post-Polio Network (www.zynet.co.uk/ott/polio/lincolnshire/), another resource for post-polio-related information.

Contact: Chris Salter, psp@loncps.demon.co.uk

 PROSTATE

listserv@listserv.acor.org

Discussion group for diseases of the prostate. The list runs on the Listserv system. On subscribing, you will be asked to confirm your intention of joining the list.

Subscribe PROSTATE Firstname Lastname

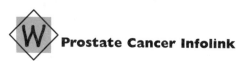 **Prostate Cancer Infolink**

www.comed.com/Prostate/

Current news, clinical reviews, clinical trials, and FAQs on prostate cancer.

Contact: webmaster@comed.com

 PSYCHIATRIC NURSING

mailbase@mailbase.ac.uk

Discussion group for nurses working in the specialty of psychiatry. The list runs on the mailbase system. On subscribing, you will be asked to confirm your intention of joining the list.

Join PSYCHIATRIC-NURSING Firstname Lastname

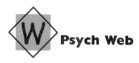 **Psych Web**

www.psychwww.com

This page contains links to sites providing information and help about specific disorders related to psychology. In addition to this page, Psych Web maintains lists of brochures and articles related to psychology (many of which are related to self-help issues), commercial psychology-related sites on the Web, other megalists of psychology resources, and scholarly psychology resources on the Web.

Contact: Russ Dewey, rdewey@gasou.edu

 Pub Manual FAQ

www.apa.org/journals/faq.html

Frequently asked questions for documenting in APA style, prepared by the staff at the American Psychological Association.

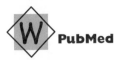 **PubMed**

www.ncbi.nlm.nih.gov/PubMed/

PubMed is the National Library of Medicine's search service that provides access to over 10 million citations in MEDLINE, PreMEDLINE, and other related databases, with links to participating online journals.

Contact: pubmednew@ncbi.nlm.nih.gov

 RARE-DIS

listserv@maelstrom.stjohns.edu

Discussion group of rare diseases. The list runs on the Listserv system. On subscribing, you will be asked to confirm your intention of joining the list.

Subscribe RARE-DIS Firstname Lastname

 Registered Nurses Association of British Columbia

www.rnabc.bc.ca/

The Registered Nurses Association of British Columbia (RNABC) is the professional organization of all registered nurses and licensed graduate nurses in the province. Everyone wishing to practice as a registered nurse in British Columbia must be a member of the association. Founded in 1912, RNABC's mandate is to serve and protect the public.

 RENALPRO

Majordomo@majordomo.srv.ualberta.ca

Discussion list for health professionals interested in topics related to nephrology and transplantation. This list runs on the Majordomo system. On subscribing, you will be asked to confirm your intention of joining the list.

Subscribe Renalpro (Note: do not include your name or e-mail address!)

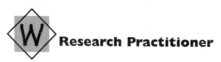 **Research Practitioner**

www.researchpractice.com

Research Practitioner is a journal published six times a year to meet the continuing education needs of research practitioners responsible for the conduct of clinical studies. This site hosts the archived articles from the journal and provides practical information that can be put to use in the day-to-day activities of clinical trials management.

Contact: info@ccrp.com

 Resources for Nurses and Families

http://pegasus.cc.ucf.edu/~wink/home.html

Resources for families, nurses, and nurse educators. Maintained by Dr. Diane Wink at the University of Central Florida.

Contact: Diane Wink, RNP, ARNP, wink@pegasus.cc.ucf.edu

 Reuters Health Information

www.reutershealth.com

Reuters Health Information Inc. produces health and medical global daily news services that keep both professionals and consumers abreast of breaking news stories in healthcare. The site also includes a searchable database of drug monographs.

Contact: webmaster@reutershealth.com

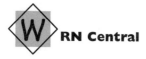 **RN Central**

www.rncentral.com

A place where nurses gather on the Web. Bulletin boards, chat rooms, and resources for students are available at this site.

Contact: Fran Beall, RN, CS, franbeall@aol.com

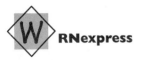 **RNexpress**

www.rnexpress.com

Online test preparation for the NCLEX-RN examination, from Springhouse Corporation. The site allows you to take a practice test on the Web (for a fee) and receive an analysis of your results.

Contact: support@rnexpress.com

 RNMGR

rnmgr-request@med-employ.com

Discussion group for nurse managers. On subscribing, you will be automatically added to the list.

Subscribe

 Robert Wood Johnson Foundation

www.rwjf.org

This site provides information about the Robert Wood Johnson Foundation, the nation's largest private philanthropy devoted to health care, its programs, and its projects, as well as information about the healthcare system. Funding information, including listings of current calls for proposals, open grants, and guidelines for grant applicants, is also available.

Contact: mail@rwjf.org

 Roxane Pain Institute

http://pain.roxane.com

This page is sponsored by Roxane Laboratories. The site includes several helpful resources related to pain management including The Shaare Zadek Cancer Pain and Palliative Care Reference Database. It also includes a complete index to and back issues of the *Palliative Care Letter*, an educational publication with abstracts of articles from scientific publications.

Contact: RPleditor@roxane.com

Royal Windsor Society for Nursing Research

www.windsor.igs.net/~nhodgins/

"Nurses enhancing nursing research at the global level through Internet technology." This Website offers a wealth of information for the novice as well as the experienced nurse researcher, including online workshops, an index of research institutions and conferences, an extensive and current database of author information for nursing journals, and a research terminology glossary. For fun, check out the retro-research (anecdotes from earlier times) and the healthcare research Jeopardy challenge.

Contact: research-nurses@canada.com

 Rural Information Center Health Service

www.nal.usda.gov/ric/richs/

The Rural Information Center Health Service (RICHS) is a joint project of the Office of Rural Health Policy, Department of Health and Human Services, and the National Agricultural Library (NAL), United States Department of Agriculture. RICHS users gain access to a national collection of rural health resources and free customized assistance online. RICHS addresses issues common to rural areas such as recruitment and retention of healthcare personnel, programs for special populations, facilities administration, network development, and innovative service delivery.

Contact: ric@nal.usda.gov

 RuralNursing

Ruralnursing-request@usask.ca

Discussion group for rural nursing. You will be subscribed automatically without a confirmation request.

Subscribe ruralnursing-l

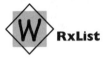 **Rush University College of Nursing**

www.rushu.rush.edu/nursing/

This site provides information on programs within the college, admissions, and organizations.

Contact: CONinfo@rushu.rush.edu

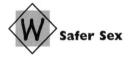 **RxList**

www.rxlist.com

A searchable database of drugs and pharmaceuticals. Search by keyword or imprint code. The site also includes the top 200 prescriptions by year (Premarin was #1 in 1999).

Contact: info@rxlist.com

 Safer Sex

www.safersex.org

Resource information on safe sex, sexuality, and health. Includes counselor resources.

Contact: info@safersex.org

 Saskatchewan Registered Nurses' Association

www.srna.org

The Saskatchewan Registered Nurses' Association (SRNA), established in 1917 by provincial legislation, is the professional, self-regulatory body for the province's 9,000 nurses. The Registered Nurses Act (1988) describes the SRNA's mandate in setting standards of education and practice for the profession and registering nurses to ensure competent nursing care for the Canadian public.

Contact: info@srna.org

SCHLRN-L

listserv@listserv.acsu.buffalo.edu

Discussion group for school nurses. The list runs on the Listserv system. On subscribing, you will be asked to confirm your intention of joining the list.

Subscribe SCHLRN-L Firstname Lastname

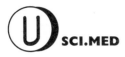 **SCI.MED**

The Usenet groups that start with "sci.med" tend to be discussions among health professionals about various health and medical diseases and specialties. Some of the sci.med Usenet groups discuss AIDS, cardiology, amyotrophic lateral sclerosis (ALS), cancer, hepatitis, Lyme disease, orthopedics, and benign prostatic hypertrophy.

 SERVICE-DOGS

Majordomo@acpub.duke.edu

Discussion group about guide, hearing, and assistance dogs. The list runs on the Majordomo system. Requests to join are forwarded to the list owner for approval. Once approved, you will be automatically added to the list.

Subscribe SERVICE-DOGS

 Shape Up America!

www.shapeup.org

This Website has been designed to provide the latest information on safe weight management and physical fitness. It includes a cyberkitchen, BMI lab (to calculate body mass index), health and fitness information, and resources designed for professionals.

Contact: suainfo@shapeup.org

Sigma Theta Tau International Nursing Honor Society

www.nursingsociety.org

Visitors to Sigma's Website can learn about the Society, obtain news on members and on the organization, access research and publications including the *Online Journal of Knowledge Synthesis for Nursing*, use the Virginia Henderson International Nursing Library, and link to chapter Websites.

Contact: stti@stti.iupui.edu

 Sinclair School of Nursing

www.muhealth.org/~nursing/docs/sonhome.html

Sinclair's Website has academic program information, a history of the University of Missouri and the school of nursing, and faculty profiles. Visitors can link to the Lottes Health Sciences Library and find out about the distance education program.

Contact: litwiller@missouri.edu

 Slack Incorporated

www.slackinc.com

Website of Slack Incorporated publishers. It contains descriptions and excerpts from books, abstracts from its journals, membership services, and public information offerings from client associations.

Contact: webmaster@slackinc.com

 Sleep Medicine Home Page

www.users.cloud9.net/~thorpy/

This Website lists extensive resources regarding all aspects of sleep, including the physiology of sleep, clinical sleep medicine, sleep research, federal and state information, patient information, and business-related groups.

Contact: thorpy@aecom.yu.edu

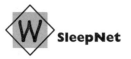 **SleepNet**

www.sleepnet.com

One objective of the SleepNet is to link all known sleep information on the Internet together at one location for easy access. Most answers to questions brought up by this Website can be found on one of the more than 50 links to sleep disorder research centers, support groups, and other organizations devoted to sleep disorders. As they say, "Everything you wanted to know about sleep disorders but were too tired to ask."

Contact: sandman@sleepnet.com

 SNURSE-L

listserv@listserv.acsu.buffalo.edu

Discussion group for nursing students. The list runs on the Listserv system. On subscribing, you will be asked to confirm your intention of joining the list.

Subscribe SNURSE-L Firstname Lastname

 Society of Pediatric Nurses

www.pednurse.org

Website for the society, with membership information, position statements, standards, and more.

 SpringNet

www.springnet.com

Website of Springhouse Corporation publishers. Visitors to this site can enjoy a wealth of information, including CE offerings, articles, news, a reference library, and career opportunities. There is a wound care center and discussion groups for nurses, nurse managers, nursing students, nurse practitioners, and emergency nurses.

Contact: e-mail directly from the site

St. Louis University School of Nursing

www.slu.edu/colleges/NR/

In addition to general information about courses and faculty, this site includes information about the nurse practitioner online distance learning program, as well as online undergraduate and graduate courses.

 Stanford Health Pages

http://stanford.thehealthpages.com

Health Pages is an online consumer healthcare service. It publishes reader-friendly information on general healthcare topics and community-specific comparative information on physicians, hospitals, allied health professionals and health plans. Consumers can search a national database of over 500,000 physicians and compare doctors in any specialty according to their experience, hospital affiliations, office services, and fees. Health Pages also incorporates the provider directories of over 300 managed care plans into a physician superdirectory, which allows consumers to determine the plans with which each provider is affiliated. There is a library of articles on such topics as prostate cancer, managed care, Medigap insurance policies, weight loss centers, and maternity care.

Contact: stanforduniversity@thehealthpages.com

 Sudden Infant Death Syndrome and Other Infant Death (SIDS/OID) Information Web Site

http://sids-network.org

This site is the growing collaborative effort of individuals from across the United States and around the world. This site offers up-to-date information, discussion groups, and data, as well as support for those who have been touched by the tragedy of SIDS/OID.

Contact: Chuck Milhalko, sidsnet@sids-network.org

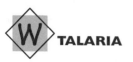 **TALARIA**

www.talaria.org

Talaria, a resource for healthcare professionals, addresses the management of pain in patients with cancer. It provides a hypermedia implementation of the AHCPR Clinical Practice Guidelines for cancer pain. Talaria provides interactive tools for healthcare providers to assist with managing pain in cancer patients, including a calculator for converting drug dosages, and an interactive dermatome map. Talaria also provides multimedia instructional tools. These include video clips of pain experts and cancer patients addressing issues regarding pain management in patients with cancer. Also included are animated tutorials on the neurological processes involved in pain and the complete text of *Current and Emerging Issues in Cancer Pain: Research and Practice.* Additional resources will be added as they become available.

Contact: bradshaw@statsci.com

 Telemedicine Information Exchange

http://tie.telemed.org/

The Telemedicine Information Exchange was created and is maintained by the Telemedicine Research Center with major support from the National Library of Medicine. TIE is a comprehensive, international, quality-filtered resource for information about telemedicine and telemedicine-related activities.

Contact: tie@telemed.org

 Texas A&M University Corpus Christi School of Nursing

www.sci.tamucc.edu/nursing/

Information on courses, programs, and faculty (including areas of research) in the School of Nursing.

Texas Nurses' Association

www.texasnurses.org

Website of the Texas Nurses' Association, with membership information, continuing education, legislative news, a members-only chat room, and consumer tips.

Contact: tna@texasnurses.org

 Texas Tech University Health Sciences Center School of Nursing

www.nursing.ttuhsc.edu

The Texas Tech School of Nursing was founded in 1981 on the Lubbock campus and expanded to Odessa, Texas, in 1985. The Texas Tech University Health Sciences Center was established in 1971 to serve the citizens of West Texas. This Web page has connections to academic program information, the Nursing Now Newsletter, faculty, advisory committees, and links to nursing Websites.

Contact: Shelley Burson, sonszb@ttuhsc.edu

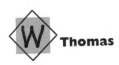 **Thomas**

http://thomas.loc.gov

Legislative information on the Internet, a service of the U.S. Library of Congress.

 Touched by a Nurse

www.touchedbyanurse.com

The lessons nurses can share are powerful, universal, and classic. These are stories have value for everyone, illustrating the power of the intense healing connections that occur because of nursing. These lessons promote a collective for the essential role nurses fill in health care. Touched by a Nurse invites you to read and share the nursing experience.

Contact: Jim Kane, tban@san.rr.com

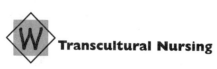 **Transcultural Nursing**

www.megalink.net/~vic/index.html

"We wish to share with nurses and other healthcare professionals our experiences and thoughts concerning the complexities involved in caring for people from diverse cultural backgrounds. Our hope is to give you some idea of the range of cultural behaviors and the need to understand people's actions from their own cultural perspective."

Contact: vic@megalink.net

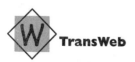 **TransWeb**

www.transweb.org

This site offers insight into organ donation and transplantation. TransWeb features news; a Top 10 Myths quiz; a multimedia guide to the transplant process; a multimedia feature called *The Transplant Journey*, which takes you on a trip through the transplant process; a focus on transplant patients; FAQs; links to other transplant resources; and information for healthcare providers. You can link to the International Transplant Nurses Society from the site (www.itns.org).

Contact: transweb@umich.edu

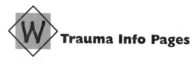 **Trauma Info Pages**

www.trauma-pages.com

Trauma Info Pages focus primarily on emotional trauma and traumatic stress, including post-traumatic stress disorder (PTSD), whether following individual traumatic experiences or a large-scale disaster. New information is added once or twice a month. The purpose of this site is to provide information about traumatic stress for clinicians and researchers in the field.

Contact: David Baldwin, PhD, dvb@trauma-pages.com

TRNSPLNT

listserv@wuvmd.wustl.edu

A discussion group related to organ transplantation and related issues. The list runs on the Listserv system. On subscribing, you will be asked to confirm your intention of joining the list.

Subscribe TRNSPLNT Firstname Lastname

 UCLA School of Nursing

www.nursing.ucla.edu/son

Information about the University of California, Los Angeles School of Nursing, a leading school of nursing in the United States. The school enjoys a national and international reputation for excellence in teaching, research, and clinical practice. There is a useful listing of ongoing faculty research.

Contact: James Kimmick, jkimmick@sonnet.ucla.edu

 UMass Graduate School of Nursing

www.umassmed.edu/gsn/

The graduate school of nursing, which offers master's and doctoral degrees, educates clinical nurse specialists and nurse practitioners within two specialties: adult acute or critical care nurse practitioner, and adult ambulatory or community care nurse practitioner. This site provides information on these programs.

Contact: Elizabeth Flodin, elizabeth.flodin@umassmed.edu

 UnCover Database of CARL

http://uncweb.carl.org

UnCover is an online periodical article delivery service and a current awareness alerting service. UnCover indexes 18,000 English language periodicals in its database and is still growing. More than 8 million articles are available through a simple online order system. Five thousand citations are added daily. Articles appear in UnCover at the same time the periodical issue is delivered to your library or local newsstand, which makes UnCover the most up-to-date index anywhere. There is no fee to search the database, but you will be charged for articles you order.

Contact: uncover@carl.org

 Uniformed Services University of the Health Sciences

www.usuhs.mil/

The Uniformed Services University of the Health Sciences (USUHS) is the nation's federal health sciences university and is committed to excellence in military medicine and public health during peace and war. USUHS provides the nation with health professionals dedicated to career service in the Department of Defense and the United States Public Health Service and with scientists who serve the common good. It serves the uniformed services and the nation as an outstanding academic health sciences center with a worldwide perspective for education, research, service, and consultation; it is unique in relating these activities to military medicine, disaster medicine, and military medical readiness. This site has information on the programs within USUHS, including the graduate school of nursing.

Contact: webmaster@usuhs.mil

 United Network for Organ Sharing

www.unos.org

Website for United Network for Organ Sharing (UNOS), the organization that administers the Organ Procurement and Transplantation Network. The site includes transplantation statistics, updated weekly.

Contact: webmaster@unos.org

 United Nurses of Alberta

www.una.ab.ca

United Nurses of Alberta (UNA) is a trade union that has represented nurses in Alberta for more than 20 years and has been instrumental in advancing the profession of nursing. UNA represents 18,000 registered nurses, registered psychiatric nurses, and mental health workers.

Contact: nurses@unab.ab.ca

 University of Akron College of Nursing

www.uakron.edu/nursing/

This Website has information on the academic program, facilities, international nursing courses, and positions available at the college of nursing. It also includes The Comfort Line, a section devoted to the concept of comfort in nursing practice and research, and The Empowerment Zone, information for advocates and healthcare professional who provide care to women experiencing domestic violence.

Contact: Linda Burr, lburr1@uakron.edu

 University of Alabama at Birmingham School of Nursing

www.uab.edu/son/

Website to introduce the school of nursing, with faculty, course listings, research activities, and more.

Contact: lrcbob@uab.edu

 University of Arizona College of Nursing

www.nursing.arizona.edu/

The University of Arizona College of Nursing Website has academic program information, research and scholarship opportunities, and faculty profiles. Visitors can also learn about computer resources and continuing education.

Contact: thompson@nursing.arizona.edu

University of Arkansas for Medical Sciences College of Nursing

www.uams.edu/nursing/

This site has information on the academic program, continuing education, faculty publications, and a history of the college of nursing. The site has a "virtual tour" of the college of nursing.

Contact: mcclainmaryf@exchange.uams.edu

 University of California, San Francisco School of Nursing

http://nurseweb.ucsf.edu/

Over 500 students enroll each year (from every continent, nation, and region) in the University of California, San Francisco (UCSF) School of Nursing master's and doctoral programs. The UCSF Nurseweb has information on these programs, the university, news, and employment. A nice, lively site with a variety of information.

Contact: data@nursing.ucsf.edu

 University of Central Florida School of Nursing

www.cohpa.ucf.edu/nursing/

This site offers information on programs, admissions, and the campus. It also has a collection of resources to other nursing Internet sites.

Contact: e-mail directly from the site

 University of Colorado School of Nursing

http://freenet.uchsc.edu/son/

The pace-setting school of nursing is known for pioneering and ongoing efforts in outreach, particularly in the MS, ND, and PhD Programs to meet rural, regional, and national healthcare needs. The school is creating an environment that shifts from the traditional faculty-student relations to one in which the student is a partner-colleague in the teaching/learning process. The school and faculty have a reputation for theory-based research, particularly in the areas of pain, rural health, migrant health, and pediatric nursing. If you link back to the UCHSC Website, you can connect to the Visible Human Project.

Contact: webadmin@freenet.uchsc.edu

 University of Connecticut School of Nursing

www.nursing.uconn.edu

This site has information on the programs within the school of nursing, the faculty, and the center for nursing research. Cybertutorials offer online readings on mastering the Internet from Susan Sparks at the National Library of Medicine.

Contact: Peggy Chinn, plchinn@uconnvm.uconn.edu

 University of Illinois at Chicago College of Nursing

www.nurs.uic.edu

Information on the college and its programs, including a useful listing of faculty and research interests.

Contact: con-help@uic.edu

 University of Iowa College of Nursing

http://coninfo.nursing.uiowa.edu

Website for the University of Iowa College of Nursing. The research section has excellent links to a variety of projects that are ongoing in the college of nursing, including the Center for Nursing Classification, Family Involvement in Care Studies, Gerontological Nursing Interventions Research Center, and more.

Contact: juanita-strait@uiowa.edu

 University of Kansas School of Nursing

http://www2.kumc.edu/son/

The University of Kansas School of Nursing offers a comprehensive curriculum that prepares students for a career in nursing at all levels. The school is known for excellence in critical care, community nursing, and advanced practice nursing, as well as thriving research and diversity programs. This site has links to the virtual classroom and distance learning at The University of Kansas Medical Center.

Contact: soninfo@kumc.edu

 University of Kentucky College of Nursing

www.mc.uky.edu/Nursing/

Information on courses, programs, and faculty in the college of nursing. There is a list of faculty research interests and doctoral dissertation titles of their graduates.

Contact: Brenda Ghaelian, brenda@pop.uky.edu

 University of Louisville School of Nursing

www.louisville.edu/nursing/

Information on courses, programs, and faculty in the school of nursing. There is a useful list of faculty research interests. On the opening page of the Website is a lovely mosaic representing nursing. Click on it to learn more about its history and meaning.

Contact: e-mail directly from the site

 University of Maine School of Nursing

www.umaine.edu/nursing/

Information on the school of nursing, faculty, courses, and programs. Link from here to the Interdisciplinary Training for Healthcare for Rural Areas (ITHCRA) Project electronic classroom.

Contact: nursing@maine.edu

University of Maryland at Baltimore School of Nursing

www.nursing.umaryland.edu

The University of Maryland School of Nursing has been a leader in merging technology into nursing learning environments, such as critical care simulation laboratories and interactive laser disc computer simulations. New to the site is Epipen: Rescue 911, an interactive computer-aided instruction program to help elementary school teachers recognize the signs and symptoms of an allergic emergency.

Contact: e-mail directly from the site

 University of Michigan School of Nursing

www.umich.edu/~nursing/

Visitors to this Website can read a message from the dean; get information on upcoming events, financial aid, and scholarships; and connect to alumni, faculty, research, and program information. There is also a link to Nursing-HealthWeb from this site.

Contact: e-mail directly from the site

 University of Minnesota School of Nursing

www.nursing.umn.edu/

The University of Minnesota School of Nursing was established in 1909 as the first continuing university-based school of nursing in the United States. It is part of the university's Academic Health Center, which is dedicated to the improvement of health through the discovery and dissemination of new knowledge. This Website has information on degree programs, the faculty, administrators, and current research.

Contact: wiebe001@tc.umn.edu

University of Nebraska Medical Center College of Nursing

www.unmc.edu/c_nursing/

At the University of Nebraska Medical Center College of Nursing site, you will find information on courses, programs, and online continuing education.

Contact: csidell@mail.unmc.edu

University of New Hampshire Department of Nursing

http://unhinfo.unh.edu/nursing/

Website for the University of New Hampshire (UNH) Department of Nursing. Program curricula, course syllabi, and faculty appointments are available at the site.

Contact: sehart@christa.unh.edu

University of North Carolina at Chapel Hill School of Nursing

www.unc.edu/depts/nursing/

This site includes information on the school of nursing and its programs. In addition, there is a nice description of the Center for Research on Chronic Illness, as well as specific research studies.

Contact: kjmorgan@email.unc.edu

University of North Carolina at Greensboro School of Nursing

www.uncg.edu/nur/

The University of North Carolina at Greensboro School of Nursing Website provides information about University of North Carolina at Greensboro (UNCG) School of Nursing programs. The site also includes useful guides to nursing resources on the Internet.

Contact: Ann Martin, ann_martin@uncg.edu

University of Pennsylvania School of Nursing

www.upenn.edu/nursing/

"These are exciting times for the University of Pennsylvania School of Nursing and the discipline of nursing. In this present ferment in health care, the opportunities for applying nursing science to advance health care are boundless. Through this Website we hope to provide a quick but thorough look at the University of Pennsylvania School of Nursing and the students—past and present—faculty, and staff who are changing the face of health care for the 21st century."

Contact: nsgweb@pobox.upenn.edu

 University of Phoenix

www.phoenix.edu

University of Phoenix offers graduate and undergraduate degree programs to working professionals around the world. With campuses and learning centers located throughout the United States and the Commonwealth of Puerto Rico, including the Online Degree Program and Center for Distance Education, University of Phoenix is one of the nation's largest private accredited institutions for business and management. This site provides information on its nursing programs, as well as many others.

Contact: e-mail directly from the site

 University of Pittsburgh School of Nursing

www.nursing.pitt.edu

Information on the educational programs within the school of nursing are contained at this site.

Contact: sjoh@pitt.edu

University of Rochester School of Nursing

www.urmc.rochester.edu/son/

This site provides an overview of the school of nursing and its academic programs.

Contact: e-mail directly from the site

 University of South Carolina College of Nursing

www.sc.edu/nursing/

The college of nursing Web page has information on departments, programs, projects, student information, faculty and staff, and distance education.

Contact: ann.lyness@sc.edu

 University of Southern Maine College of Nursing and Health Professions

www.usm.maine.edu/~son/

Information on the college of nursing and health professions, the faculty, courses, and programs.

Contact: con@usm.maine.edu

 University of Tennessee at Chattanooga School of Nursing

www.utc.edu/~utcnurse/

Information on the programs and courses are available at this site. There is a handy listing of faculty, including expertise, research interests, and teaching areas. In addition, Web projects by students in the MSN program are highlighted.

Contact: Pam Taylor, RN, PhD, Pam-Taylor@utc.edu

University of Texas at Austin School of Nursing

www.utexas.edu/nursing

This site has detailed information on the programs, courses, and faculty at the school of nursing. It also includes abstracts of current faculty research.

Contact: beckstein@mail.utexas.edu

 University of Texas Health Science Center at San Antonio

www.nursing.uthscsa.edu

"Welcome to our School of Nursing, one of five schools at the Health Science Center at San Antonio. The others include the School of Allied Health Sciences, School of Medicine, Dental School, and the Graduate School of Biomedical Sciences. The School of Nursing offers a Bachelor of Science in Nursing degree (BSN), a Master of Science in Nursing degree (MSN) and a Doctor of Philosophy degree (PhD) in nursing. There are accelerated BSN and MSN programs for LVNs and RNs. The University of Texas Health Science Center at San Antonio School of Nursing celebrates its 30 year anniversary in 1999, having graduated over 6,000 students."

Contact: Elaine Graveley, DBA, RN, graveley@uthscsa.edu

 University of Texas-Galveston School of Nursing

www.son.utmb.edu

This site includes information on the school of nursing, its programs, faculty, students, and research. There are some interesting historic pictures of the university and Galveston.

Contact: plrichar@utmb.edu

 University of Texas-Houston School of Nursing

http://sonser4.nur.uth.tmc.edu

This site includes information on the school of nursing, its programs, faculty, students, and research. Links to the UT-Houston Center on Aging.

University of Texas M.D. Anderson Cancer Center

www.mdanderson.org

This site contains extensive information and resources for cancer care from the renowned M.D. Anderson Cancer Center, the Texas Cancer Data Center, and CancerNet.

Contact: e-mail directly from the site

 University of Utah College of Nursing

www.nurs.utah.edu/

The nursing program at the University of Utah became a college of nursing in 1948, awarding the baccalaureate degree to both generic and registered nurse students. The baccalaureate and graduate programs are fully accredited by the National League for Nursing. The college is the only PhD nursing program in the state of Utah to prepare nursing faculty. This Website details these programs.

Contact: webmaster@nurs.utah.edu

 University of Virginia School of Nursing

www.nursing.virginia.edu

This Website contains academic program information, descriptions of the research and academic centers, faculty profiles, and links to other nursing Internet resources.

Contact: nur-webmaster@virginia.edu

 University of Washington School of Nursing

www.son.washington.edu/

The University of Washington School of Nursing has been ranked #1 in the United States since 1984. This site has academic program information and connects to the school's three departments: Biobehavioral Nursing and Health Systems, Family and Child Nursing, Psychosocial and Community Health. If you connect to the main Website of the university (www.washington.edu), you will see a live picture of the campus—on sunny days, you can see Mt. Rainier in the background!

Contact: ahale@u.washington.edu

 University of Wisconsin-Madison School of Nursing

www.son.wisc.edu/~son/

This site includes information on faculty, courses, and programs within the school of nursing. There are narrative descriptions of faculty research and interests, as well as a nursing museum on the site. Within the museum, the Caps Collection includes donations from the alumni of nearly 100 schools of nursing.

Contact: lhdore@facstaff.wisc.edu

 University of Wisconsin-Milwaukee School of Nursing

www.uwm.edu/Dept/Nursing/

"As the premier urban research university in Wisconsin, UW-Milwaukee is an institution committed to active engagement with our community partners in meeting the challenges of urban life. Through the expansion of existing programs and the development and implementation of new collaborative projects sponsored through the Milwaukee Idea Initiative begun in 1998, the School of Nursing is providing active leadership in this important and progressive effort. Please take the time to visit our Web pages and learn more about our Institute for Urban Health Partnerships, our four community nursing centers, the Center for Cultural Diversity and Health, the Historical Gallery and our Health Careers Bridge Program."

Contact: asknursing@csd.uwm.edu

 U.S. Department of Health and Human Services

www.dhhs.gov

Information about the mission of the U.S. Department of Health and Human Services (HHS), plus HHS publications and press releases and links to other government health and medicine resources on the Internet.

Contact: e-mail directly from the site

U.S. News and World Report Graduate School Rankings

www.usnews.com/usnews/edu/beyond/bcheal.htm

Each year, U.S. News and World Report, Inc. ranks nursing graduate schools overall and by program. Rankings in the health professions are based on the results of surveys sent to deans, faculty, and administrators of accredited graduate programs, who assess the quality of curriculum, faculty, and graduates.

 ## U.S. Pharmacopeia

www.usp.org

The U.S. Pharmacopeia sets the standards that manufacturers must meet to sell their products in the United States.

Contact: webmaster@usp.org

 ## Vaccine Research, National Institute of Allergy and Infectious Diseases

www.niaid.nih.gov/publications/vaccine.htm

The site contains fact sheets and brochures, news releases, and links on vaccines.

Contact: e-mail directly from the site

 ## Vanderbilt University School of Nursing

www.mc.vanderbilt.edu/nursing/

With a history dating back to 1909, Vanderbilt University School of Nursing has an established reputation for excellence in nursing education. This Website has information on academics, faculty projects on the Web, research, and the Nashville community.

Contact: webmaster@mcmail.vanderbilt.edu

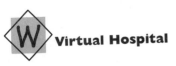 Virtual Hospital

http://vh.radiology.uiowa.edu/

The Virtual Hospital is a digital health sciences library created in 1992 at the University of Iowa to help meet the information needs of healthcare providers and patients. The goal of the Virtual Hospital digital library is to make the Internet a useful medical reference and health promotion tool for healthcare providers and patients. The Virtual Hospital digital library contains hundreds of books and brochures for healthcare providers and patients.

Contact: librarian@vh.org

 Virtual Nursing Center

http://www-sci.lib.uci.edu/HSG/Nursing.html

Martindale's Health Science Guide links to nursing resources such as medical dictionaries and glossaries, metabolic pathways and genetic maps, interactive anatomy browsers, online nursing journals, nurses' courses, tutorials and lectures, interactive patient browsers, and general nursing information.

Contact: Jim Martindale, jmartindale@hotbot.com

 Virtual Nursing College

www.langara.bc.ca/vnc/

The Virtual Nursing College (VNC) is a virtual learning and teaching environment that uses concept-resource mapping, multimedia, and full access to Internet and virtual reality. This page offers a comprehensive list of links to nursing research resources, cardiovascular information, pharmacology and drug resources, publications, nursing terminology and nursing data sets information, and holistic sites.

Contact: Jack Yensen, jyensen@langara.bc.ca

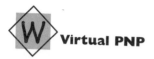 **Virtual PNP**

http://home.earthlink.net/~emgoodman/virtualpnp.htm

A Website for pediatric nurse practitioners and their child and adolescent patients. The site includes case studies, clinical insights, professional links, employment opportunities, and continuing education.

Contact: Eric Goodman, MSN, emgoodman@earthlink.net

 Visiting Nurse Associations of America

www.vnaa.org

Today, visiting nurse agencies (VNAs) care for nearly 10 million people every year, and represent nearly one-quarter of all not-for-profit, freestanding home healthcare services in the United States. The Website offers information for care-givers, help locating a VNA, and links to home care resources.

Contact: vnaa@vnaa.org

 Wayne State University College of Nursing

www.nursing.wayne.edu

Information on the college of nursing, its programs, courses, and faculty. There is an interesting and detailed description of the Center for Health Research.

Contact: nursinginfo@wayne.edu

 Web of Addictions

www.well.com/user/woa/

The Web of Addictions is dedicated to providing accurate information about alcohol and other drug addictions. It provides a resource for teachers, students, and others who needed factual information about abused drugs.

Contact: Andrew L. Homer, ahomer@mail.coin.missouri.edu

Web Extension to American Psychological Association Style

www.nyct.net/~beads/weapas/

For those of you writing term papers or manuscripts for publication, here is the source that tells you how to document your online references in proper APA style.

Contact: webmaster@beadsland.com

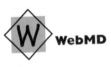 ## WebMD

www.webmd.com

WebMD is an Internet healthcare company connecting physicians and consumers to each other and to the healthcare community. Its vision is to improve health and wellness around the world by using the Internet to facilitate a new system for the delivery of health care. The result is a single environment for communications and transactions among physicians, consumers, and healthcare institutions.

Contact: Andrew L. Homer, ahomer@mail.coin.missouri.edu

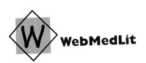 ## WebMedLit

www.webmedlit.com

WebMedLit is a medical headlines service. WebMedLit scans the Web each night for journal citations and abstracts. All links point back to the original articles or abstracts at the publishers' Websites. In general, the sources followed must provide at least some abstracts to the full-text articles; sites providing only tables of contents are not tracked by WebMedLit. The sources tracked by WebMedLit are primarily concerned with clinical topics or human epidemiology. The site is sponsored by Silver Platter Information, Inc.

Contact: feedback@webmedlit.com

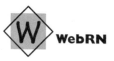 **WebRN**

www.webrn.com

WebRN includes breaking healthcare and nursing news; industry forums and discussion groups for issues and trends; online continuing education and personal log books; patient education, including online, interactive teaching tools; clinical references; a career center; e-mail; and professional supplies.

Contact: nursing@webmd.net

 Wellness Web

http://wellweb.com

A resource for healthcare consumers, with health education information on topics ranging from smoking to heart disease to women's health. For a quick guide to the material available at the site, choose the alphabetical Master Index from the main menu.

Contact: wellness@wellweb.com

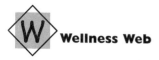 **WellTech International**

www.welltech.com

The WellTech site is designed to provide online resources for health promotion and wellness professionals. WellTech gathers, develops, and manages health promotion resources from around the world. WellTech's goal is to link health educators, wellness directors, publishers, and health program developers with the information critical to their work.

Contact: info@welltech.com

 West Virginia University School of Nursing

www.hsc.wvu.edu/son/

Website for school of nursing at WVU. Information on the North Central West Virginia "Nursing Workforce Network" is contained at this site.

Contact: drichter@wvuson1.hsc.wvu.edu

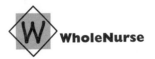 **WholeNurse**

www.wholenurse.com

Information on complementary therapies, cultural issues, and what's happening in the holistic community.

Contact: webmaster@nurseportal.com

 Wisconsin Geriatric Education Center

www.marquette.edu/wgec/

The ultimate goal of the Wisconsin Geriatric Education Center (WGEC) is to enhance the quality of life and promote wellness for the elderly in Wisconsin through the stimulation, coordination, implementation, and dissemination of geriatric education for healthcare faculty and providers. This site provides a variety of information toward accomplishing that goal.

Contact: wgecnet@marquette.edu

 Wisconsin Nurses' Association

www.wisconsinnurses.com/

Website of the Wisconsin Nurses' Association, with membership information, STAT bulletins, a nurse practitioner forum, advanced practice forums, and more.

Contact: wna@execpc.com

 WITSENDO

listserv@listserv.dartmouth.edu

Discussion group on endometriosis.

Subscribe WITSENDO Lastname, Firstname

WOMENS-HEALTH-NETWORK

Majordomo@coombs.anu.edu.au

Discussion group on women's health. The list runs on the majordomo system. When you submit a request to subscribe, you will be asked to confirm your request.

Subscribe WOMENS-HEALTH-network

 World Health Organization

www.who.int/

Website of the World Health Organization, located in Geneva, Switzerland. The objective of WHO is the attainment by all peoples of the highest possible level of health. There is a wealth of information available at this site. A good search engine helps you quickly access the materials you need.

Contact: info@who.ch

Index

Note: Page numbers in *italics* indicate illustrations; those followed by t indicate tables; and those followed by d indicate display text.

227

Instructions for using *Nurses' Guide to the Internet, 3rd Edition* software

To help you use this book as efficiently as possible, the enclosed software provides direct links to each Internet address listed in the text. Using the file on the disk provided, you can easily locate all of the sites listed in the book with one click. This file will work with any Web browser.

TO USE THE ENCLOSED DISK:

1. Follow the normal steps to run the Web browser you would like to use. (Consult the main text if you need assistance setting up your Web browser.)
2. Insert the enclosed disk into your disk drive.
3. Open the floppy disk drive on your computer (usually drive A:).
4. Double-click on the file "Nurses' Guide to the Internet, 3rd edition."
5. Click on the address for any Website or mailing list you would like to access.

   Websites will open in your Web browser; mailing lists will launch and run through your e-mail software. (If you are subscribing to a mailing list, carefully note the subscription instructions.)

6. **To return to the directory list of sites, click the "back" button on your Web browser.**

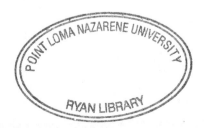